Inclusive Radiology: Fostering Diversity and Equity in Academic and non-Academic Settings

Sarah Keller-Yamamura • Jin Yamamura
Editors

Inclusive Radiology: Fostering Diversity and Equity in Academic and non-Academic Settings

Springer

Editors
Sarah Keller-Yamamura
Department of Radiology
Charité-Universitätsmedizin Berlin,
Corporate Member of Freie Universität
Berlin and Humboldt-Universität zu Berlin
Berlin, Germany

Jin Yamamura
Department of Diagnostic and
Interventional Radiology and Nuclear
Medicine
University Medical Center Hamburg-
Eppendorf (UKE)
Hamburg, Germany

ISBN 978-3-032-05704-4 ISBN 978-3-032-05705-1 (eBook)
https://doi.org/10.1007/978-3-032-05705-1

This Springer imprint is published by the registered company Springer Nature Switzerland AG
The registered company address is: Gewerbestrasse 11, 6330 Cham, Switzerland

Contents

About the Editors

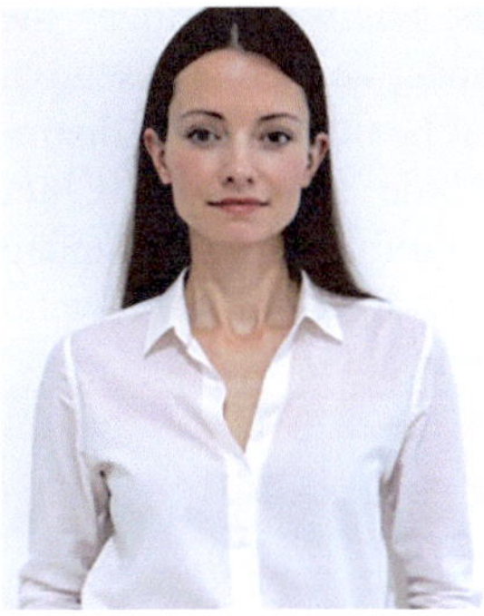

Sarah Keller-Yamamura is a consultant in radiology and private lecturer at Charité-Universitätsmedizin Berlin. She holds a master's degree (MPH) in Global Public Health from Imperial College London, with a focus on digital health, health economics, and epidemiology. Her academic and research interests span clinical and preclinical quantitative MRI as well as health systems and gender equity. As head of a Gender & Diversity research group, she focuses on structural barriers and opportunities in academic careers, scientific publishing, and the advancement of diversity in radiology and healthcare more broadly.

Sarah works in the pharmaceutical industry since 2021 and is currently active in the field of market access, where she develops evidence strategies, shapes access frameworks, and supports equitable pathways to innovation within local regulatory and legislative landscapes. She has authored and led multiple studies on gender equity and diversity in medicine and serves as an advisory board member for Women in Global Health (WGH), contributing to global efforts to promote women's leadership, career equity, and health rights.

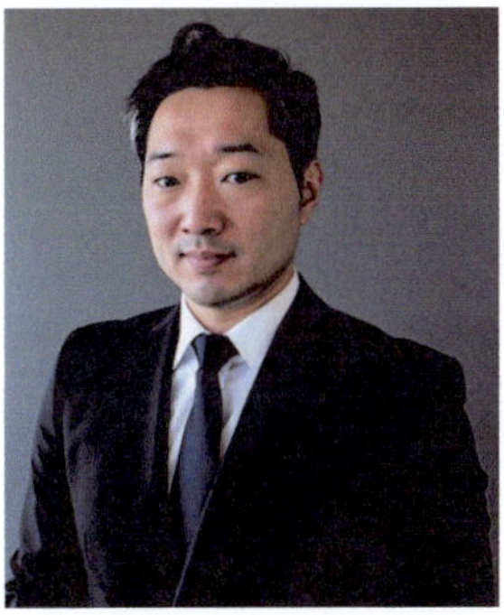

Jin Yamamura is a radiologist and professor of digital health. He holds a professorship at the University Medical Center Hamburg-Eppendorf (UKE) and was recently appointed Professor of Digital Health at IB University of Health and Social Sciences in Berlin. His academic and clinical career spans over two decades, with a focus on digital transformation, research, and innovation in radiology. He served as Director and Chairman of the Department of Diagnostic and Interventional Radiology at Immanuel Clinics Rüdersdorf-Berlin, affiliated with the Medical School

Brandenburg, where he successfully established a fully digitized radiology department. He has also worked as a Visiting Professor and Researcher in Diagnostic Radiology at Osaka University Hospital, Japan, and has authored more than 100 scientific publications.

In addition to his academic and clinical roles, he has been active in the healthcare industry since 2021. He currently serves as General Manager for Care Area & Digital Solutions, International at GE HealthCare, where he is responsible for business strategy and market development across all care areas and digital solutions outside the United States. His work bridges the intersection of clinical excellence, academic research, and digital innovation in global healthcare. His distinguished accomplishments include serving as Chief Medical Director for DeepSpin GmbH. He has founded his own ventures and held advisory roles for several companies such as NortHH Medical GmbH.

Part I

Academic Radiology and Diversity

1 Research and Publications in Diagnostic Radiology

Sarah Keller-Yamamura and Jin Yamamura

1.1 Introduction

Academic publishing is the cornerstone of career development and scientific contribution in medicine, particularly in diagnostic radiology, where technological advancements, diagnostic techniques, and innovation are rapidly evolving. Publications in peer-reviewed journals indicate scholarly productivity and measures contributing to academic recognition, funding, and promotion. In this context, the underrepresentation of women in radiology authorship has garnered attention as a potential barrier to career advancement. Despite the growing number of women in medical schools, they remain underrepresented in academic radiology, particularly in senior roles and key authorship positions. This chapter examines gender-specific disparities in diagnostic radiology publications and explores the factors contributing to and potentially alleviating this imbalance.

1.2 Authorship Representation in Academic Publications

Academic publications play a crucial role in shaping the career paths of radiologists. Numerous studies indicate that research output is a significant factor in faculty promotions, grants, and leadership roles within academic medicine. For example,

S. Keller-Yamamura (✉)
Department of Radiology, Charité-Universitätsmedizin Berlin, Corporate Member of Freie Universität Berlin and Humboldt-Universität zu Berlin, Berlin, Germany
e-mail: sarah.keller@charite.de

J. Yamamura
Department of Diagnostic and Interventional Radiology and Nuclear Medicine, University Medical Center Hamburg-Eppendorf (UKE), Hamburg, Germany
e-mail: j.yamamura@uke.de

S. Keller-Yamamura, J. Yamamura (eds.), *Inclusive Radiology: Fostering Diversity and Equity in Academic and non-Academic Settings*,
https://doi.org/10.1007/978-3-032-05705-1_1

publication metrics like the h-index, citation counts, and the roles of first and last authors are highly valued during promotions. Last, or senior, authorship often denotes leadership in research endeavors and marks academic seniority. The underrepresentation of women in these roles highlights ongoing barriers that impede their ability to achieve senior faculty positions. In the following, recently published articles on gender parity in diagnostic radiology publications have been summarized to gain a more comprehensive picture of the situation.

Nischal et al. (2022) [1] retrospectively investigated female authorship in a total of 431 musculoskeletal radiology articles across three major journals in 10-year intervals from 2000 to 2020: *Skeletal Radiology* (SR), *Clinical Radiology* (CR), and the *Indian Journal of Radiology and Imaging* (IJRI). The study showed a significant increase in female first authorship in SR (from 0.8% in 2000 to 5.4% in 2020). However, female last authorship was extremely low (0% in 2000 and 0.15% in 2020). IJRI reached a proportion of female first authors of 4.8%, but 3.2% of female last authors in 2020; however, percentages must be interpreted with care as absolute numbers were extremely small. CR displayed the lowest numbers of female first and last authorships in MSK articles (3.6% and 0% in 2020, respectively). The authors concluded that the gender gap in MSK radiology is exceptionally high, urging immediate attention to benefit patient care and institutes.

Furthermore, the authors postulated that promoting clinical staff should focus on publication metrics and involvement in patient care and clinical excellence. Comparable to Nischal et al. [1], Hsu et al. (2021) [2] explored authorship trends in *Skeletal Radiology* in the long term. From its inception in 1976 to 2020, the study noted a significant increase in female first and last authorship, with female representation in both roles rising steadily ($p = 0.02$). In more detail, female first authors contributed 0% in 1976 and grew to 37.8% in 2020; female last authors increased from 0% in 1976 to 21.2% in 2020. Besides female contribution, the number of published articles per year, coauthors per article, and affiliations per year increased significantly in the 44-year span. The study also observed a growing geographic diversity, particularly in Asian contributions, although female authorship increases were more region-specific. The authors concluded that there is a positive trend in the participation of women in authorships, even in musculoskeletal research, which is very male-dominated, giving hope for a future gender balance. It is interesting to note the discrepancy between the results and those of Nischal et al., who measured significantly lower proportions of women in *Skeletal Radiology* in 2020. The discrepancy can be explained by the fact that Nischal et al. only included assigned MSK articles and thus a significantly lower number of cases in their analyses and that this particular field differs from the general publication figures in *Skeletal Radiology*.

Molwitz et al. (2021) [3] analyzed trends in female authorship across 10 radiology journals with varying impact factors (low–medium–high). Between 2007 and 2018, female first authorship increased from 22.2% to 29.1%, while female senior authorship rose from 11.1% to 16.1%. The most significant gains were observed in low-impact journals, where female first and senior authorship doubled. The chance to publish in a low- or medium-ranked journal compared to a high-impact journal was significantly higher for women, with an adjusted Odds ratio (AOR) of 1.5 and

1.8, respectively. Among the high-impact journals, the highest publication numbers for female first authors were observed in *European Radiology* (32.4%; 95% CI [29.3–35.8]; $p < 0.0001$). Female last authors published more frequently in *Investigative Radiology* (32.4%; 95% CI [29.3–35.8]; $p < 0.0001$). Interestingly, the analysis showed that male collaboration, reflected by first and last authorships on research projects and, thus, publications, was around four times more common than female or mixed-gender collaboration. This finding aligns with various research articles postulating a need to increase mentorship, especially for aspiring female radiologists, by promoting women to senior positions where they can contribute collectively to female advancement and serve as role models for the younger generation. Other reasons for the low numbers of female authorships might be influenced by editorial board composition, where gender disparity is still a sad reality [4].

Campbell et al. (2019) [5] yielded to quantify the relationship between author gender and publication topic. The authors examined gender-specific original research articles in major radiology journals, such as *Radiology*, the *American Journal of Roentgenology*, and *Academic Radiology*, from 2011 to 2015. Data showed that women represented 30% of first and 25% of last authors. 83% of article topics were gender-neutral, 14% published in women's health, and 3% in men's health. Articles on women's health were significantly associated with female authors, with a five-fold increased likelihood of having a female first author and a 6.4-fold increase for female last authors. These articles also garnered more citations (an average of 27.6 citations) than gender-neutral articles (21.9 citations), reflecting the academic impact of gender-specific research. The authors concluded that the researcher's gender strongly influences gender-related research and positively impacts overall citation counts and rates over the year. It is questionable what these findings imply for future generations as these findings could also be influenced by the comparable lower number of overall research conducted in these narrow subspecialties. However, regarding strategic career positioning, specialization in academic radiology might be advantageous and contribute to higher achievements in h-index and subsequent career promotion.

Liang et al. (2015) [6] conducted a two-decade review of general radiology journals, analyzing 3,786 articles published between 1993 and 2013. The percentage of women as first authors increased from 19.7% in 1993 to 32.1% in 2013, while female senior authorship rose from 13.6% to 19.1%. The most significant gains were noted in journals such as the *American Journal of Roentgenology* (AJR) and *Radiology*, where female senior authorship increased by 7–11 percentage points. The authors argued with a general assumption that first authorships symbolize active participation in research projects, whereas last authorships stand for a supervising, research project leading role in academic medicine. Although the proportion of female authorship is increasing, it is still clearly lagging, especially about the last authorship, indicating that many women start a radiological academic career, for example, as part of their doctoral thesis, but do not continue this or do not rise to a leading position. The distribution of first and last authorships may be a good proxy in most cases, even if a strategic change of author positions occurs repeatedly. However, this will certainly rarely be the case.

The approach of Piper et al. (2016) [7] was slightly more specific. They performed a 35-year analysis of radiology US authorship, examining trends from 1978 to 2013. In total, 4,217 original articles and editorials displaying US first or senior authors with MD degrees were abstracted. The proportion of female first authors rose from 8.3% in 1978 to 32.4% in 2013, while female senior authorship increased from 6.8% to 21.9%. Interestingly, the number of articles authored by nonphysician female first and senior authors rose from 4% to 45.9% and 17.2% to 31.6%, respectively. Also, the study highlighted that female first authors were significantly more likely to collaborate with female senior authors. This finding has been described frequently in current literature, emphasizing the importance of mentorship networks. This aspect is interesting in that, at least in the USA, gender parity among female researchers outside the clinic is more balanced, which could indicate structural barriers that make it impossible for women in medical practice to carry out research alongside their clinical duties.

McKenzie et al. (2017) [8] conducted a more specific long-term analysis of female authorship trends in *Emergency Radiology* over the past 20 years. In total, 1617 articles were retrospectively reviewed, including original articles, case reports, review articles, and pictorial essays. Female first authorship increased from 17.5% in 1994 to 20.9% in 2014, while female last authorship rose significantly from 12.9% to 21.3%. Articles coauthored by female first and last authors also increased from 25% in 1994 to 35% in 2014, though not significantly. The findings suggest modest progress but highlight continued barriers to female leadership. The results fit well into the overall context of author trends in general diagnostic radiology. They are, therefore, more balanced than the still very unevenly distributed authorships in MSK-specific research articles. Concerning the USA, the authors again refer to the unevenly distributed workforce in the radiology clinic, with a proportion of women of approximately 27% [6]. The authors also recommend mandatory work on research projects as part of residency training to bring prospective radiologists closer to research. In the German context in particular, this approach may not necessarily be expedient, as most prospective doctors here are already involved in research, at least briefly, as part of their doctoral thesis and therefore already have a clear preference as junior doctors as to whether they prefer an academic or purely clinical career. In addition, the value of clinically excellent radiologists should not be neglected as they are very relevant for direct patient care. Therefore, career advancement should not be based solely on research performance, as Nischal et al. [1] suggested in the article described above. Concerning the US-based analysis from McKenzie et al. [8], Li et al. (2021) [9] studied trends in the *Canadian Association of Radiologists Journal* from 2010 to 2019. Female first authorship rose to 39.8%, while female last authorship reached 26.9%. Although the odds of female authorship increased, female last authorship did not strongly predict female first authorship, indicating gaps in mentorship or collaboration opportunities.

Ayyala et al. (2022) [10] devoted their analysis to author trends in pediatric radiology. They specifically examined only articles published in *Pediatric Radiology* between January 2017 and December 2020 and further limited their analysis to articles submitted from North America. To further assess the impact of the

COVID-19 pandemic on female authorship in *Pediatric Radiology*, the study team conducted quarterly comparisons between 2019 and 2020. From 2017 to 2020, female first authorship increased from 38.6% to 43.2%, but female last authorship temporarily declined during the early pandemic phase (March–May 2020), likely due to increased caregiving responsibilities. Above, female first and last authorships were significantly higher for educational articles, such as pictorial essays and reviews. The study underscores the disproportionate impact of external crises on female academics. The study thus indicates several aspects of unequal distribution; firstly, the drop in authorship in the early days of the COVID pandemic, which can serve as a proxy for structural inequality, for example, in the care of children at times of collective institutional failure such as closed daycare centers and schools, and secondly that although women are interested and eager to contribute to publications, their preference, at least in pediatric radiology in North America, is for educational articles. From a purely academic, career-oriented perspective, however, this approach may not be expedient as nonoriginal research articles are significantly less relevant in terms of achieving important academic milestones such as habilitation or associate professorships and are therefore more likely to have an unequal time/benefit ratio for the author, despite their importance for the readership.

In a very vast approach, Xiao et al. (2023) [11] reviewed 23,741 articles in the major radiology journals *Radiology, American Journal of Roentgenology, Journal of the American College of Radiology*, and *Academic Radiology* over 13 years (2007–2020). Overall, 72.4% of article authors, independently from the author's position, were male. A slight majority (54%) of articles displayed a male first and last author. Female authorship increased steadily, with women comprising 28% of first authors and 20% of senior authors by 2020. Using a statistical approach of random pairing, significantly fewer male-female author combinations and more female–female author combinations were expected ($p < 0.01$), findings that are in line with a variety of research, claiming the preference for same-gender author collaboration (and mentoring) [3]. However, female authors received fewer citations (3.2 fewer on average) than their male counterparts, suggesting persistent challenges in gaining academic recognition despite increased participation. An interesting aspect of the study is the lower rate of citations of studies published by women. This issue has already been investigated and described in previous studies [12, 13], but whether this bias is directly attributable to the name of the authors or whether other factors have an influence, for example, that the general writing style of women appeals less to men or the topics of the published research appeal to a smaller audience, has already been discussed. Double blinding of the author's gender in the review process and the editorial board has been implemented in some journals. All these and many more factors must be considered to allow a conclusion to be drawn on the results of the citation count.Table 1.1 lists an overview of studies published between 2015 and 2023 on gender trends in authorship in diagnostic radiology.

Academic publishing plays a pivotal role in shaping careers and advancing scientific contributions in diagnostic radiology, where publication metrics such as first and last authorship are critical indicators of research involvement and leadership. Several investigations reveal that while female first authorship has improved, the

Table 1.1 Selected overview of studies published between 2015 and 2023 on gender trends in authorship in diagnostic radiology

Author	Year	Journal	Medical disciplines analyzed	Title
Ayyala, R. et al.	2022	*Pediatr Radiol*	Pediatric radiology	Gender trends in the authorship of pediatric radiology publications and the impact of COVID-19 pandemic
Campbell, J. et al.	2019	*AJR Am J Roentgenol*	Radiology, women's health	Authorship and impact of gender-specific research in major radiology journals
Hsu, A. et al.	2021	*Skeletal Radiol*	Musculoskeletal (wide field) radiology	A comprehensive analysis of authorship trends in skeletal radiology since inception
Liang, T. et al.	2015	*AJR Am J Roentgenol*	Diagnostic radiology	Assessing the gap in female authorship in radiology: trends over the past two decades
Li, N. et al.	2021	*Can Assoc Radiol J*	Diagnostic radiology	Female authorship in radiology: trends in the past decade in CARJ
McKenzie, K. et al.	2017	*Emergency Radiology*	Emergency radiology	Assessing the gap in female authorship in the journal *Emergency Radiology*: trends over 20 years
Molwitz, I. et al.	2021	*Eur Radiol*	General radiology	Gender trends in authorships and publication impact in *Academic Radiology*: A 10-year perspective
Nischal, N. et al.	2022	*Clin Radiol*	Musculoskeletal radiology (very specific)	Assessing the gender gap in musculoskeletal radiology authorship across three continents
Piper, C. et al.	2016	*AJR Am J Roentgenol*	Diagnostic radiology	Gender trends in radiology authorship: a 35-year analysis
Xiao, N. et al.	2023	*Acad Radiol*	Diagnostic radiology	Gender disparities in academic radiology authorship: a 13-year review

progression to leadership positions remains slow. For instance, studies focusing on musculoskeletal radiology show only modest gains in female first authorship and extremely low figures for female senior authorship. At the same time, long-term analyses indicate regional variability and suggest that structural factors within academic medicine contribute to these imbalances.

Further research indicates that although female authorship is on the rise, women are still less likely to occupy pivotal roles in research projects, and collaborations led by male authors are more common. Specialized topics like women's health tend to have higher female representation and garner more citations. Yet, these niches may not offer the same career advancement opportunities as broader research areas. The impact of external factors, notably the COVID-19 pandemic, has also been significant, with increased caregiving responsibilities adversely affecting female senior authorship in fields like pediatric radiology. Moreover, comprehensive reviews of large datasets confirm the dominance of male authors in the literature and point to disparities in recognition, as evidenced by lower citation counts for studies authored by women.

1.3 Conclusion

While diagnostic radiology is witnessing gradual improvements in female authorship, the enduring gender disparities—especially in leadership roles—underscore the need for systemic changes. Addressing these imbalances is crucial not only for ensuring equitable career advancement but also for fostering a diverse and innovative academic environment that benefits patient care and the evolution of the discipline. Therefore, academic institutions and journals are encouraged to adopt reforms that support mentorship, recognize diverse contributions, and mitigate structural barriers, paving the way for a more balanced and inclusive future in radiological research and practice.

References

1. Nischal N, Iyengar KP, Vaishya R, Haleem S, Zaw Pe E, Choudur HN, Botchu R. Assessing the gender gap in musculoskeletal radiology authorship across three continents: are really the "ladies first"? Clin Radiol. 2022;77(10):724–9. https://doi.org/10.1016/j.crad.2022.05.030.
2. Hsu AL, Konner M, Muttreja A, Lee CH, Chien JL, Irish RD. A comprehensive analysis of authorship trends in *Skeletal Radiology* since inception from 1976 to 2020. Skeletal Radiol. 2021;50(12):2519–23. https://doi.org/10.1007/s00256-021-03810-y.
3. Molwitz I, Yamamura J, Ozga AK, Wedekind I, Nguyen TA, Wolf L, Kamo M, Zhao J, Can E, Keller S. Gender trends in authorships and publication impact in Academic Radiology-a 10-year perspective. Eur Radiol. 2021;31(12):8887–96. https://doi.org/10.1007/s00330-021-07928-4.
4. Abdellatif W, Shao M, Jalal S, et al. Novel geographic thematic study of the largest radiology societies globally: how is gender structure biased within editorial boards? AJR Am J Roentgenol. 2019; https://doi.org/10.2214/AJR.18.20965:1-6.
5. Campbell JC, Yoon SC, Grimm LJ. Authorship and impact of gender-specific research in major radiology journals. J Am Coll Radiol. 2019;16(2):240–3. https://doi.org/10.1016/j.jacr.2018.08.024.
6. Liang T, Zhang C, Khara RM, Harris AC. Assessing the gap in female authorship in radiology: trends over the past two decades. J Am Coll Radiol. 2015;12(7):735–41. https://doi.org/10.1016/j.jacr.2015.03.008.
7. Piper CL, Scheel JR, Lee CI, Forman HP. Gender trends in radiology authorship: a 35-year analysis. AJR Am J Roentgenol. 2016;206(1):3–7. https://doi.org/10.2214/AJR.15.15116.
8. McKenzie K, Ramonas M, Patlas M, Katz DS. Assessing the gap in female authorship in the journal *Emergency Radiology*: trends over a 20-year period. Emerg Radiol. 2017;24(6):641–4. https://doi.org/10.1007/s10140-017-1510-x.
9. Li N, Alabousi M, Patlas MN. Female authorship in radiology: trends in the past decade in CARJ. Can Assoc Radiol J. 2021;72(3):388–91. https://doi.org/10.1177/0846537120946641.
10. Ayyala RS, Trout AT. Gender trends in authorship of *Pediatric Radiology* publications and impact of the COVID-19 pandemic. Pediatr Radiol. 2022;52(5):868–73. https://doi.org/10.1007/s00247-021-05213-6. Epub 2021 Oct 21.

11. Xiao N, Marquez-Karry R, Oliveira DFM, Berggruen S, Horowitz JM. Gender disparities in academic radiology authorship: a 13-year review. Acad Radiol. 2023;30(8):1714–20. https://doi.org/10.1016/j.acra.2022.10.031.
12. Wenneras C, Wold A. Nepotism and sexism in peer-review. Nature. 1997;387:341–3. https://doi.org/10.1038/387341a0.
13. Caplar N, Tacchella S, Birrer S. Quantitative evaluation of gender bias in astronomical publications from citation counts. Nat Astron. 2017:1. https://doi.org/10.1038/s41550-017-0141.nEdedgaTg.

Gender Disparities in Radiology Subspecialties: Research, Academic Publications, and Opportunities for Improvement

2

Elif Can and Sarah Keller-Yamamura

2.1 Introduction

Radiology has become a cornerstone of modern medicine, revolutionizing diagnostics and treatment through technological innovation and precision medicine. Despite these advancements, the field faces persistent and significant gender disparities across its subspecialties. Women, who now represent approximately 70% of medical school graduates globally, are disproportionately underrepresented in radiology and its leadership roles [1, 2]. This discrepancy contributes to a troubling brain drain phenomenon, where highly trained female professionals migrate to other fields or step away from clinical practice altogether. Such attrition is not only a loss of talent but also a missed opportunity to foster diverse perspectives that drive innovation and improve patient care outcomes [3–5].

The challenges are multifaceted. In interventional radiology (IR), a male-dominated subspecialty, women face significant structural and cultural barriers, including implicit bias, limited mentorship, and concerns about radiation safety [6, 7]. Neuroradiology and pediatric radiology reflect similar patterns of underrepresentation in leadership, even where female participation in the workforce is relatively high [8–10]. These disparities are compounded by intersectional barriers faced by women of color, who experience both racial and gender biases, limiting their career trajectories.

E. Can
Department of Diagnostic and Interventional Radiology, Medical Center University of Freiburg, Faculty of Medicine, University of Freiburg, Freiburg, Germany
e-mail: elif.can@uniklinik-freiburg.de

S. Keller-Yamamura (✉)
Department of Radiology, Charité-Universitätsmedizin Berlin, Corporate Member of Freie Universität Berlin and Humboldt-Universität zu Berlin, Berlin, Germany
e-mail: sarah.keller@charite.de

S. Keller-Yamamura, J. Yamamura (eds.), *Inclusive Radiology: Fostering Diversity and Equity in Academic and non-Academic Settings*,
https://doi.org/10.1007/978-3-032-05705-1_2

Addressing these disparities is not simply a matter of fairness; it is a critical imperative for the future of radiology. A diverse and inclusive workforce fosters better decision-making, enhances research innovation, and improves patient care by integrating varied perspectives. This chapter examines gender disparities across key radiology subspecialties, highlights the compounding effects of intersectionality, and proposes actionable recommendations to create equitable career pathways for all radiologists [1, 6, 8, 10, 11].

2.2 Gender Disparities Across Subspecialties

2.2.1 Interventional Radiology (IR)

Interventional radiology (IR) is among the most innovative branches of radiology. It specializes in minimally invasive procedures guided by imaging technologies. Despite its groundbreaking contributions to modern medicine, IR remains a male-dominated field. Morgan et al. (2024) found that only 12–16% of trainees in IR are women [12]. Parvataneni et al. (2025) found that women represent only 9.9% of interventional radiologists in the United States, with gender bias (OR 12.13, $p < 0.001$) and work–life balance concerns identified as primary deterrents [6]. The study also highlighted that limited professional advancement opportunities (OR 0.56, $p = 0.006$) significantly impact female participation. Their findings underscore the importance of mentorship programs, flexible training pathways, and addressing implicit bias in recruitment. The underrepresentation extends beyond demographics to research and leadership, where female professionals face limited opportunities to secure grants, present at conferences, and assume prominent academic roles. Female researchers in IR frequently report fewer opportunities for mentorship and professional visibility compared to their male colleagues [6, 13]. Blum et al. (2024) observed that female interventional radiologists in Germany were significantly underrepresented in academic roles, holding only 29% of research positions. Women also reported feeling less recognized at professional congresses (53% vs. 93% of men) and faced reduced confidence in their professional networks. The authors recommend initiatives such as protected research time and tailored mentorship to improve female representation in IR [13, 14]. Theodoulou et al. (2022) found that differences in motivation factors for pursuing a career in interventional radiology (IR) revealed notable gender-specific variations. Mentoring was identified as a significant factor for 8.7% of female respondents compared to 21.6% of male respondents. Similarly, the influence of senior colleagues was more prominent among men, with 25.0% citing it as a key factor, compared to 15.2% of women. Despite these differences, the majority of participants, regardless of gender, strongly agreed or agreed that early exposure to IR training in the first year of medical studies had a positive impact on their decision to pursue a career in IR, with 82.6% of women and 81.3% of men endorsing this view [7]. Parvataneni et al. (2025) identify several key deterrents to women pursuing IR careers. Gender-related bias was cited as a major barrier, with an odds ratio of 12.13, indicating a strong association between perceived bias and reduced interest among women. Concerns about work–life balance, the ability to become pregnant, and limited opportunities for professional advancement further exacerbate these disparities. Goswami et al. (2022) revealed that women accounted for only 12.1% of academic interventional radiologists, with even fewer in executive roles. Despite having comparable years of practice and research output, women face systemic barriers to leadership, pointing to the need for structural reforms and equitable evaluation criteria [9]. Wang et al. (2019) also examined gender distribution in publications and research activities within the Society of Interventional Radiology (SIR). They found that the proportion of female first authors in the *Journal of Vascular and Interventional Radiology* (JVIR) increased from 10% in 2008 to 14.6% in 2018 ($p = 0.01$). Similarly, the proportion of female senior (last) authors rose from 7.1% to 11.9% over the same period ($p = 0.006$). At the editorial level, the proportion of women on the JVIR editorial board grew from 5.4% in 2008 to 14.3% in 2018 ($p = 0.002$). Additionally, the share of female authors in *IR Quarterly* increased from 4.5% in 2012 to 27% in 2018 ($p = 0.02$). These findings demonstrate progress in female representation in publications and editorial roles, though women remain underrepresented, particularly in senior research position [15]. Malhotra et al. (2023) identified intersectional inequities in IR, where Asian women earned 15% less than white men in similar positions. The study highlights the compounded effects of race and gender bias on compensation and advancement, advocating for policy-level interventions to address pay disparities [16]. Addressing these disparities requires targeted interventions. Radiation safety education programs are essential to dispelling myths and encouraging more women to enter the field [6, 17–19]. A lot of studies suggest that addressing implicit biases and creating structured support systems will be crucial for retaining women in IR [6, 12–14, 17, 20–22].

2.2.2 Neuroradiology

Neuroradiology, a subspecialty dedicated to diagnosing and treating conditions affecting the nervous system, highlights some of the most significant gender disparities in radiology. Ahmadi et al. (2018) report that women hold only 12.5% of leadership positions in neuroradiology, despite comprising 25% of assistant professors. Male faculty members have a significantly higher median H-index (17.5) compared to their female counterparts, reflecting disparities in research productivity. This imbalance limits women's opportunities for career advancement and perpetuates systemic inequities [8]. Structural and cultural barriers compound these challenges. Female professionals are underrepresented in senior authorship roles and on editorial boards, reducing their academic visibility [23]. Lack of mentorship opportunities further hinders the career progression of women in neuroradiology, creating a cycle of underrepresentation [2, 21, 23–25].

Singhal and Aiken (2022) noted that the "motherhood penalty" disproportionately affects female neuroradiologists, limiting their promotion and retention. The authors recommend institutional policies such as flexible work arrangements and structured mentorship programs to support women balancing professional and family responsibilities [23]. Goswami et al. (2022) found that women constituted only 22.8% of academic neuroradiologists, with significant disparities in attaining professorships and executive roles. These findings call for systemic changes in academic evaluation criteria and increased diversity in leadership selection [9]. Nguyen et al. (2023) state that gender disparities in neurology authorship positions are stark, with women representing only 24.6% of last authors and 36.2% of first authors between 2002 and 2020. The study emphasizes that such disparities not only hinder the career advancement of women but also limit the diversity of perspectives in academic literature, which is crucial for driving innovation and scientific rigor. Additionally, the tendency of male last authors to collaborate more frequently with male first authors perpetuates these disparities, underscoring the need for systemic changes to improve equity in authorship and mentorship opportunities [26]. Efforts to address these disparities must focus on increasing female representation in authorship and editorial roles. Leadership development programs that provide training in grant writing, networking, and academic career planning can equip women with the tools they need to excel [8]. Collaborative mentorship initiatives, involving both male and female mentors, are also crucial for bridging gaps in guidance and support, fostering an inclusive environment that drives innovation and improves patient care.

2.2.3 Breast Imaging

Breast imaging is one of the few radiology subspecialties where women constitute the majority, representing 69% of practitioners [1]. Seely et al. (2024) reported that while women dominate breast imaging (79.1% of practitioners), only 58.3% hold leadership positions. Factors such as part-time work (27% of women vs. 9% of men) and institutional biases in promotions contribute to this disparity. The authors recommend leadership training programs and institutional reforms to bridge the gender gap in decision-making roles [1]. Nguyen et al. (2022) emphasized that despite the high representation of women in breast imaging, systemic academic biases persist, limiting women's access to funding and high-impact publications [24] similar to others [27, 28]. They suggest equity-focused mentorship programs to ensure balanced career progression and research representation [24].

Haken et al. (2021) highlighted the underrepresentation of women in senior leadership roles in breast imaging, with less than 10% serving as department chairs. The study argues for comprehensive mentorship initiatives and implicit bias training to promote equity in leadership opportunities and improve outcomes for underserved populations [29]. Seely et al. (2024) and Halley et al. (2018) highlight that systemic biases and organizational barriers often exclude part-time practitioners from leadership pathways [1, 30]. Additionally, challenges in accessing professional development opportunities and securing equitable promotions persist. Despite these barriers, breast imaging has pioneered initiatives such as mentorship programs and flexible work policies that foster gender equity. Further efforts are needed to address persistent inequities. Expanding leadership pathways to include part-time practitioners and implementing transparent promotion criteria are essential steps. These measures can ensure that opportunities in breast imaging are based on merit rather than schedules, allowing women to advance their careers and continue to serve as role models for gender equity across radiology subspecialties.

2.2.4 Pediatric Radiology

Pediatric radiology stands out for its relatively high representation of women, who account for 45% of the workforce. However, this representation does not extend to leadership roles, where women remain underrepresented. Nearly half of the women entering this field face significant life events, such as childbirth, during their training or early careers, underscoring the need for supportive institutional policies [1, 10, 11, 30]. AAP Policy Statement (2013) emphasized the need for equitable parental leave policies, recommending at least 6–8 weeks of paid leave for residents. Such policies are vital for retaining female practitioners and enabling career progression without penalization for life events like childbirth [10]. The barriers in pediatric radiology include biases against women in decision-making roles and limited access to mentorship opportunities [29]. These challenges are compounded by the lack of comprehensive parental leave policies and support systems for balancing career and family responsibilities [1]. Addressing these disparities requires targeted measures to create a more inclusive environment for female professionals.

Fishman et al. (2021) analyzed authorship trends in three high-impact pediatric journals from 2001 to 2016 and observed a notable increase in female representation among both first and senior authors. Female first authorship rose from 39.8% to 57.7%, while senior authorship increased from 28.6% to 38.1% during the study period. Despite these gains, women remained underrepresented in senior authorship and editorial board roles, with female representation on editorial boards growing from 17.8% in 2001 to 39.8% in 2016. The study also found that junior female faculty were more likely to co-author with senior women rather than senior men, a trend that may hinder opportunities for career advancement given existing gender disparities in leadership and promotion [31]. Böhme et al. (2022) conducted a comprehensive bibliometric analysis of 156,642 pediatric research articles, revealing that while women account for 46.6% of all authorships, they are underrepresented in prestigious positions such as last authorships, with a Prestige Index of −0.13. Despite an increasing proportion of female authors over time (from 42.5% in 2008 to 49.9% in 2018), significant gender disparities persist, particularly in leadership and senior authorship roles. The study highlights the "leaking pipeline," where many women leave academic pediatrics before reaching senior positions, often due to lifestyle priorities and a lack of role models. Encouragingly, projections suggest a narrowing gender gap, with female authors potentially surpassing gender neutrality in prestigious authorships by 2023. This underscores the need for targeted interventions to ensure women are equitably represented in leadership within pediatric research [32]. Cohen et al. (2021) examined pediatric chair turnover and demographics across US medical schools, finding that while the proportion of female chairs has increased from 5.5% in 1980 to 40% in 2020, women remain underrepresented relative to their overall presence in the pediatric faculty (26.3% of chairs vs. 60% of faculty). The study highlights that Black and Hispanic chairs, while proportionate to their representation among pediatric faculty, remain underrepresented compared to their proportions in the US population. Additionally, chair retention varied across time periods, with the median tenure declining from 10 years before 1985 to 7 years in more recent cohorts. The increasing number of interim chair appointments, now comprising 40% of new chairs in Pediatrics, may impact strategic continuity and leadership development within departments. The authors advocate for intentional efforts to diversify the leadership pipeline to address persistent inequities in representation and tenure [33]. Equitable parental leave policies and robust return-to-work programs can provide crucial support for women during life transitions. Mentorship and peer support networks can offer valuable guidance, helping women navigate the challenges of balancing professional and personal responsibilities [34]. Increasing the visibility of successful female leaders in pediatric radiology can inspire the next generation and promote greater gender equity in the field [1–3, 8, 11, 18, 35–38].

2.2.5 Conclusion

Despite persistent gender disparities in academic roles and publications within radiology, there are promising signs of gradual improvement. In neuroradiology, while women remain underrepresented in leadership and authorship, studies have documented incremental progress, particularly in female first and middle authorship. Nguyen et al. (2023) reported that the proportion of female first authors across neurology-related fields increased from 26.3% in 2002 to 37.4% by 2020, signaling a positive trend in early-career academic opportunities for women. Although last authorship remains predominantly male, the rise in first authorship positions indicates that more women are entering the academic publishing pipeline. In breast imaging, where women represent the majority of practitioners, leadership roles have become more accessible, with women holding 58.3% of decision-making positions. Pediatric radiology has similarly witnessed gains, with first authorship by women rising from 39.8% to 57.7% over a 15-year period, along with increased senior authorship. Publications in interventional radiology show progress as well, with female first authorship in the *Journal of Vascular and Interventional Radiology* increasing from 10% in 2008 to 14.6% in 2018, and the proportion of female editorial board members expanding during the same period. These developments, while modest, reflect the impact of targeted initiatives such as mentorship programs, equity-driven policies, and flexible career pathways. Continued efforts to address systemic barriers and promote inclusivity will be essential to sustaining and accelerating these positive trends, ensuring a more equitable future for women in radiology.

2.3 General Recommendations Across Subspecialties

Efforts to address gender disparities and workforce attrition in radiology must focus on creating a sustainable and inclusive environment that retains talent and fosters equity. Below are targeted recommendations to address these challenges. Radiology must actively engage female medical students early in their education. Radiology subspecialties must adopt comprehensive strategies to address gender disparities and promote equity. Early exposure to radiology during medical training, coupled with diverse role models, can inspire interest among female students [12, 13, 17–19, 22]. Implicit bias training programs can raise awareness and mitigate unconscious biases in hiring, promotions, and grant evaluations. Targeted grants and fellowships for women can boost their research contributions and academic visibility [39, 40]. Despite the growing proportion of female medical graduates, many opt out of radiology due to misperceptions of the field, lack of role models, and concerns about lifestyle balance. Different authors reported that early exposure to radiology, particularly in subspecialties like interventional radiology, increased interest by over 50% [7, 12, 17]. Recruiting women into the field requires not only educational outreach but also visible representation of diverse professionals in leadership and clinical roles [1, 2, 35, 41]. Mentorship remains one of the most effective tools for advancing gender equity. However, mentorship must also account for intersectionality, recognizing that women of color face compounded challenges [2, 21, 24, 25, 42]. Tailored mentorship programs, such as those integrating cultural competency and addressing systemic racism, can provide critical guidance for underrepresented groups. Sponsorship, which involves senior professionals actively advocating for mentees, must be expanded to support diverse candidates for leadership and academic roles [25]. Retention strategies are essential to counteract the brain drain observed among female radiologists. A significant portion of women leave radiology due to work-life balance issues, lack of support during parental leave, and stagnant career progression [1, 30]. Providing flexible work schedules, on-site childcare, and equitable parental leave policies—such as those recommended by the American Academy of Pediatrics (AAP)—can mitigate these challenges [10]. Additionally, institutions should track the career trajectories of radiology graduates to identify patterns of attrition and implement targeted retention programs. Compensation inequities remain a critical barrier for women in radiology. Malhotra et al. (2023) identified a 15% pay gap between Asian women and white male radiologists in equivalent roles, with similar disparities observed across other intersectional identities [16]. Transparent salary audits and equitable promotion criteria must be institutional priorities. Creating clear pathways for part-time practitioners to access leadership roles ensures that career advancement is based on merit rather than rigid schedules.

Radiology societies and institutions must prioritize leadership training for women, focusing on skills such as strategic planning, negotiation, and academic visibility. Expanding opportunities for women to serve on editorial boards, grant review panels, and conference committees can increase their influence in shaping the field. Seely et al. (2024) emphasized that achieving equity in leadership is essential for fostering inclusive decision-making and innovation in patient care [1]. Implicit biases in hiring, evaluations, and mentorship contribute to systemic barriers for women and underrepresented minorities. Regular, mandatory bias training for all radiology staff can raise awareness and promote equity [1, 35, 43]. However, cultural change must go beyond training, with senior leadership modeling inclusive behaviors and holding institutions accountable for diversity metrics [21, 44–48]. Institutions must adopt data-driven approaches to understand why women leave radiology. Tracking metrics such as gender representation across career stages, retention rates, and exit interviews can provide valuable insights. This data should inform policy decisions, such as improving work-life integration or addressing barriers to leadership for women and underrepresented groups [9, 44]. Intersectional challenges amplify the barriers faced by women of color in radiology. Nguyen et al. (2022) observed that Black and Hispanic women reported significantly lower publication rates than their peers, a gap attributed to systemic biases and limited mentorship opportunities [24]. Institutions must implement programs specifically designed to address the unique needs of these groups, such as targeted research funding and tailored mentorship initiatives [49]. Women in radiology are underrepresented in grant awards and high-impact publications [50, 51]. Targeted research funding, equitable distribution of research responsibilities, and transparent grant application processes are essential. Institutions must also recognize and reward diverse forms of academic contributions, ensuring that women's research efforts are equally valued. Professional societies can play a vital role in fostering collaborative networks for women in radiology. Creating platforms for peer mentorship, knowledge sharing, and advocacy can strengthen career development and amplify the voices of underrepresented groups. These networks can also serve as incubators for innovative research and inclusive policies.

2.4 Conclusion of Recommendations

Achieving gender equity in radiology is a multifaceted challenge that requires systemic reforms, cultural shifts, and intentional investment in talent retention. By addressing gender disparities and intersectional barriers, radiology can transform into a model of inclusivity that enhances innovation, collaboration, and patient care. These recommendations provide a framework for institutions to build a sustainable and equitable future for radiologists, ensuring that no talent is left behind.

References

1. Seely JM. Women in radiology: challenges and opportunities. J Breast Imaging. 2024;6(5):539–46.
2. Kubik-Huch RA, Vilgrain V, Krestin GP, Reiser MF, Attenberger UI, Muellner AU, et al. Women in radiology: gender diversity is not a metric-it is a tool for excellence. Eur Radiol. 2020;30(3):1644–52.

3. Fichera G, Busch IM, Rimondini M, Motta R, Giraudo C. Is empowerment of female radiologists still needed? Findings of a systematic review. Int J Environ Res Public Health. 2021;18(4):1542.
4. Cater SW, Yoon SC, Lowell DA, Campbell JC, Sulioti G, Qin R, et al. Bridging the gap: identifying global trends in gender disparity among the radiology physician workforce. Acad Radiol. 2018;25(8):1052–61.
5. Tsugawa Y, Jena AB, Figueroa JF, Orav EJ, Blumenthal DM, Jha AK. Comparison of hospital mortality and readmission rates for medicare patients treated by male vs female physicians. JAMA Intern Med. 2017;177(2):206–13.
6. Parvataneni K, Tamposi R, Mercaldo N, Englander MJ, Josephs S, Uceda M, et al. What deters women from pursuing careers in interventional radiology: factors associated with medical trainees decisions to pursue careers in IR. Curr Probl Diagn Radiol. 2025;54(1):70–4.
7. Theodoulou I, Dost S, Burrows V, Lyall F, Wah TM, Makris GC. The interventional radiology gender gap: perspectives from the international IR training survey. Br J Radiol. 2022;95(1136):20210726.
8. Ahmadi M, Khurshid K, Sanelli PC, Jalal S, Chahal T, Norbash A, et al. Influences for gender disparity in academic neuroradiology. AJNR Am J Neuroradiol. 2018;39(1):18–23.
9. Goswami AK, Kokabi N, Khaja MS, Saad WE, Khaja A, Vashi AP, et al. Academic radiology in the United States: defining gender disparities in faculty leadership and academic rank. Acad Radiol. 2022;29(5):714–25.
10. Section on Medical Students Rs, and Fellowship Trainees, Childhood CoE. Parental leave for residents and pediatric training programs. Pediatrics. 2013;131(2):387–90.
11. Morgan JC, Owens T, Carmack MC, Braverman A, Class QA. Policy and perceptions of pregnancy during training among residents of various subspecialties. Postgrad Med J. 2024;101:441.
12. Morgan RA, Patel PJ, Binkert C, Tam A, (SIR) CaIRSoECatSoIR. Global statement defining interventional radiology-have we reached the tipping point? J Vasc Interv Radiol. 2024;47:1433.
13. Blum SFU, Dewald CLA, Becker L, Staudacher E, Franke M, Katoh M, et al. The status of academic interventional radiologists in Germany with focus on gender disparity: how can we do better? CVIR Endovasc. 2024;7(1):47.
14. Dewald CLA, Blum SFU, Becker LS, Barzakova E, Franke M, Westphalen K, et al. Exploring gender roles in German interventional radiology – how progressive are we? Rofo. 2024;197:814.
15. Wang M, Laguna B, Koethe Y, Lehrman E, Kumar V, Kohi MP. Bridging the gender gap in the society of IR: a benchmark study. J Vasc Interv Radiol. 2019;30(4):584–8.e2.
16. Malhotra A, Futela D, Khunte M, Wu X, Payabvash S, Gandhi D, et al. Intersectionality and faculty compensation in academic radiology in U.S. Acad Radiol. 2024;31(12):5228–31.
17. Cao Y, Yu L, Xiong F, Wang J, Kan X, Zheng C. Longitudinal investigation of undergraduates' radiation anxiety, interest, and career intention in interventional radiology. Eur Radiol. 2024;34(12):7797–803.
18. Lightfoote JB, Fielding JR, Deville C, Gunderman RB, Morgan GN, Pandharipande PV, et al. Improving diversity, inclusion, and representation in radiology and radiation oncology part 1: why these matter. J Am Coll Radiol. 2014;11(7):673–80.
19. Can E. From fear to fascination: transforming interest in interventional radiology. Eur Radiol. 2024;34(12):7795–6.
20. Ullrich L, Uller W, Frisch A. [Interventional radiology – training and career opportunities]. Radiologie (Heidelb). 2024.
21. Li S, Sun VH, Galla N, Salazar G, Lewis T, Ahmed M, et al. Gender-based survey analysis of research and mentoring in interventional radiology. J Vasc Interv Radiol. 2022;33(5):578–85.e3.
22. Snyder A, Xiang D, Smith A, Esswein S, Toubat O, Di Capua J, et al. Gender disparities among medical students choosing to pursue careers in medical research: a secondary cross-sectional cohort analysis. BMC Med Educ. 2021;21(1):591.
23. Singhal A, Aiken A. Call to action: women in neuroradiology's group (WINNERS)-is there a need? AJNR Am J Neuroradiol. 2022;43(10):1396–9.

24. Nguyen M, Chaudhry SI, Asabor E, Desai MM, Lett E, Cavazos JE, et al. Variation in research experiences and publications during medical school by sex and race and ethnicity. JAMA Netw Open. 2022;5(10):e2238520.
25. Deitte LA, McGinty GB, Canon CL, Omary RA, Johnson PT, Slanetz PJ. Shifting from mentorship to sponsorship-a game changer! J Am Coll Radiol. 2019;16(4 Pt A):498–500.
26. Nguyen AX, Yoffe L, Li A, Trinh XV, Kurian J, Moss HE, et al. Gender gap in neurology research authorship (1946-2020). Front Neurol. 2021;12:715428.
27. Giannotti E, Clauser P, van Nijnatten TJA, Schiaffino S. Gender gap among authorships of artificial intelligence articles in breast imaging. Eur J Radiol. 2024;180:111691.
28. Shawn Yuan PH, Yan TD, Sharma S, Chahley E, MacLean LJ, Freitas V, et al. Authorship gender among articles about artificial intelligence in breast imaging. Eur J Radiol. 2024;175:111428.
29. Haken OJ, Gong AJ, Ambinder EB, Myers KS, Oluyemi ET. Diversity and inclusion in breast imaging and radiology at large: what Can we do to improve? Curr Radiol Rep. 2021;9(12):13.
30. Halley MC, Rustagi AS, Torres JS, Linos E, Plaut V, Mangurian C, et al. Physician mothers' experience of workplace discrimination: a qualitative analysis. BMJ. 2018;363:k4926.
31. Fishman M, Williams WA, Goodman DM, Ross LF. Gender differences in the authorship of original research in pediatric journals, 2001-2016. J Pediatr. 2017;191:244–9.e1.
32. Böhme K, Klingelhöfer D, Groneberg DA, Bendels MHK. Gender disparities in pediatric research: a descriptive bibliometric study on scientific authorships. Pediatr Res. 2022;92(1):80–90.
33. Cohen MB, Aban I, Artman M, Binney G, Blake A, Boney C, et al. Pediatric chair turnover and demographics. J Pediatr. 2022;242:4–7.e3.
34. Company M. Unlocking the full potential of women at work United States: McKinsey & Company; 2012 [Available from: https://www.mckinsey.com/capabilities/people-and-organizational-performance/our-insights/unlocking-the-full-potential-of-women-at-work.
35. Martinez NE. Women in radiation: a brief discussion of the intersectionality of race and gender. J Radiol Prot. 2021;41(3):590.
36. Shore LM, Chung BG. Inclusion as a multi-level concept. Curr Opin Psychol. 2024;60:101910.
37. Sepulveda KA, Paladin AM, Rawson JV. Gender diversity in academic radiology departments: barriers and best practices to optimizing inclusion and developing women leaders. Acad Radiol. 2018;25(5):556–60.
38. Lee D, Jalal S, Nasrullah M, Ding J, Sanelli P, Khosa F. Gender disparity in academic rank and productivity among public health physician faculty in North America. Cureus. 2020;12(6):e8553.
39. Jena AB, Olenski AR, Blumenthal DM. Sex differences in physician salary in US Public Medical Schools. JAMA Intern Med. 2016;176(9):1294–304.
40. Xiao N, Marquez-Karry R, Oliveira DFM, Berggruen S, Horowitz JM. Gender disparities in academic radiology authorship: a 13-year review. Acad Radiol. 2023;30(8):1714–20.
41. Martinez S, Araj J, Reid S, Rodriguez J, Nguyen M, Pinto DB, et al. Allyship in residency: an introductory module on Medical Allyship for Graduate Medical Trainees. MedEdPORTAL. 2021;17:11200.
42. Scammell JM, Olumide G. Racism and the mentor-student relationship: nurse education through a white lens. Nurse Educ Today. 2012;32(5):545–50.
43. Liang R, Dornan T, Nestel D. Why do women leave surgical training? A qualitative and feminist study. Lancet. 2019;393(10171):541–9.
44. Battaglia F, Farhan SA, Narmeen M, Karimuddin AA, Jalal S, Tse M, et al. Does gender influence leadership roles in academic surgery in The United States of America? A cross-sectional study. Int J Surg. 2020;83:67–74.
45. Grimm LJ, Lowell DA, Cater SW, Yoon SC. Differential motivations for pursuing diagnostic radiology by gender: implications for residency recruitment. Acad Radiol. 2017;24(10):1312–7.
46. Wang Y, Li J, Ou-Yang X, Wan M, Zhang G, Yi H. Bridging the gap: advancing gender equality in medical research. Postgrad Med J. 2024;101:670.

47. Hamed S, Thapar-Björkert S, Bradby H, Ahlberg BM. Racism in European health care: structural violence and beyond. Qual Health Res. 2020;30(11):1662–73.
48. Gopal DP, Rao M. Playing hide and seek with structural racism. BMJ. 2021;373:n988.
49. Hattery AJ, Smith E, Magnuson S, Monterrosa A, Kafonek K, Shaw C, Mhonde RD, Kanewske LC. Diversity, equity, and inclusion in research teams: the good, the bad, and the ugly. In: Race and Justice. SAGE Publications; 2022. p. 505–30.
50. Molwitz I, Yamamura J, Ozga AK, Wedekind I, Nguyen TA, Wolf L, et al. Gender trends in authorships and publication impact in academic radiology-a 10-year perspective. Eur Radiol. 2021;31(12):8887–96.
51. Yamamura J, Molwitz I, Ozga AK, Nguyen TA, Wedekind I, Wolf-Baldauf L, et al. Gender differences and cooperation in medical authorships – an analysis of the recent ten years in five key medical disciplines. BMC Med Educ. 2023;23(1):68.

Research and Publications: Do Interdisciplinary Differences Exist?

3

Sarah Keller-Yamamura and Jin Yamamura

3.1 Introduction

The research contributions of its members significantly shape the advancement of academic medicine. Publications and authorship in peer-reviewed journals serve as key indicators of academic productivity and are often linked to career advancement, recognition, and leadership opportunities. Although gender equality in medical education has notably improved over the past few decades, disparities persist in academic authorship, especially at senior levels. These disparities affect not only individual researchers' careers but also the diversity and breadth of scientific inquiry.

Academic authorship plays a critical role in shaping the discourse and direction of medical research. The opportunity to publish and lead research projects often correlates with greater professional visibility, funding opportunities, and leadership roles within the field. However, systemic barriers, biases, and structural challenges have limited equitable access to these opportunities, especially for women and other underrepresented groups in academia. Understanding the scope and scale of these disparities is essential to identify actionable strategies for fostering inclusivity.

This chapter focuses on whether interdisciplinary differences exist in gender equality in research and publications, specifically focusing on radiology compared to other medical disciplines. It explores trends in authorship, the barriers that

S. Keller-Yamamura (✉)
Department of Radiology, Charité-Universitätsmedizin Berlin, Corporate Member of Freie Universität Berlin and Humboldt-Universität zu Berlin, Berlin, Germany
e-mail: sarah.keller@charite.de

J. Yamamura
Department of Diagnostic and Interventional Radiology and Nuclear Medicine, University Medical Center Hamburg-Eppendorf (UKE), Hamburg, Germany
e-mail: j.yamamura@uke.de

S. Keller-Yamamura, J. Yamamura (eds.), *Inclusive Radiology: Fostering Diversity and Equity in Academic and non-Academic Settings*,
https://doi.org/10.1007/978-3-032-05705-1_3

prevent equal representation, and lessons that can be learned from fields that have achieved more significant gender equity. By examining these issues through a comparative lens, the chapter aims to highlight actionable insights for addressing inequities in academic medicine.

3.2 Gender Equality in Research and Publications

Radiology, as a field, has seen an incremental rise in female representation in research authorship. However, this progress has been uneven and limited in certain areas. According to Huang et al. [1], female first authorship in radiology journals grew from 13.0% in 1984 to 31.5% in 2014, while senior authorship increased from 9.3% to 22.1% during the same period. These figures demonstrate a positive trajectory and highlight a significant senior-level underrepresentation. Subspecialties within radiology reveal further disparities. For example, breast imaging exhibits higher rates of female authorship, with first authorship reaching 48.3% compared to technical-focused papers, where female first authorship was as low as 5.5%. This suggests that subspecialties with higher female physician representation tend to have more gender-balanced research contributions. Another issue is the citation gap. Huang et al. [1] noted that articles authored by women were less frequently cited than those by men, though the gap has narrowed over time. The reduced visibility of female-led research can impact recognition and opportunities for career advancement, further perpetuating gender inequities.

The landscape of gender equality in authorship varies significantly across medical disciplines, with some fields showing progress while others lag behind. For example, Gadek et al. [2] investigated authorship trends in the *Journal of Perinatology* during the COVID-19 pandemic compared to the previous 15-month period and found that women made up 62% of first authors and 53% of overall authors, reflecting the high proportion of female practitioners in neonatology. However, only 43% of last authors were women, revealing ongoing disparities at senior levels [2]. Elias et al. analyzed gender equity in COVID-19-related publications across four high-impact general medicine journals and two hospital medicine-focused journals. Women accounted for 34% of authorship credits overall, and 43% in hospital medicine-specific journals. Disparities were even more apparent in general medicine journals, where women hospitalists earned only 26.3% of author credits [3].

Rubulotta et al. [4] provided insights into internal medicine societies. 76% of the surveyed societies' presidents were men, while 20% were women. Australia showed the highest percentage of women board presidents, and the lowest proportion was found in Europe and Asia. The proportion of board members was barely higher, with 27% women. This imbalance is reflected by the overall proportion of women first authors in high-impact internal medicine journals (impact factor > 10), where women represented less than 40% [5]. Networking and structural factors, such as the organization of conferences and societal norms, were identified as significant barriers to equitable authorship and leadership opportunities.

Beland et al. [6] cross-sectionally analyzed trends in urology publications in 2019 in five journals with the highest urological impact and found that women comprised 22.1% of first authors and 14.6% of senior authors, significantly exceeding their workforce representation of 9.9%. Despite this, urology remains one of the most gender-imbalanced fields in terms of academic leadership and senior authorship, with women comprising only 4.5% of chair positions in urology compared to 14% of department chairs across other medical specialties [7].

A study comparing authorship across various clinical disciplines was published by Jagsi et al. in 2006 [8]. The authors documented a 35-year analysis of gender gaps in leading medical journals, revealing that the percentage of female first authors increased from 5.9% in 1970 to 29.3% in 2004, while senior authorship rose from 3.7% to 19.3%. The most significant gains were observed in pediatrics and obstetrics, whereas fields like surgery showed minimal improvement, with senior authorship for women remaining below 7%. Despite an increase in the proportion of female physicians in many fields, this has not consistently resulted in equal representation in authorship. Yamamura et al. [9] analyzed the ratio of female physicians to female authorship in radiology, urology, surgery, gynecology, and pediatrics across the United States, Canada, the United Kingdom, France, Germany, and Japan over a decade (2007/8 to 2017/18). They discovered that pediatrics and gynecology, where over 50% of physicians are female, exhibited balanced or higher female first authorship in relation to their workforce proportion. In contrast, radiology lagged behind, with 23.4% of physicians being female in 2017/18, reflecting a similar proportion of female first authorship. Surgery displayed the greatest disparity, with women comprising 13% of surgeons but only 11.9% of senior authors in surgical research. This gap highlights systemic barriers preventing female physicians from advancing to senior academic roles, even in fields where they are well-represented at entry levels.

In clinical oncology, Hornstein et al. [10] conducted a cross-sectional study on authorships in the *Journal of Clinical Oncology Global Oncology* from its inception in 2015 to March 2020, revealing stark gender inequities, particularly in low-income regions such as sub-Saharan Africa and South Asia, where women constituted only 21.6% of first authors and 9.1% of last authors. Among these, sub-Saharan Africa (18.8%) and South Asia (14.5%) had the lowest proportions of female last authors. In contrast, female first authors contributed a greater proportion than males in Europe, Central Asia, and North America. Categorized by the World Bank's designations for the fiscal year 2020, female first authors accounted for a higher proportion than males in high-income countries (HIC) and upper-middle-income countries (UMIC). However, they showed significant underrepresentation in low-income countries (LIC) and low-middle-income countries (LMIC). In terms of last authors, females were significantly underrepresented across all economic areas. Notably, articles with female last authors were significantly more likely to also have female first authors (odds ratio 2.2, 95% confidence interval 1.6–3.2) and to have 50% or more female co-authors (odds ratio 1.4, 95% confidence interval 0.9–2.1), underscoring the importance of mentorship and leadership diversity.

Ghattas et al. [11] examined trends in 26 US-based orthopedic journals between 2002 and 2021 and found that while female first authorship increased significantly over 20 years to 13.6%, last authorship saw a more modest rise to just 9.9%. Also, in orthopedics, articles with female first authors were significantly more likely to feature female last authors (odds ratio 2.22; 95% confidence interval 2.1–2.4), suggesting the importance of collaborative female mentorship in advancing representation.

In ophthalmology, Fathy et al. [12] investigated authorships in three major ophthalmologic journals between 2005–9 and 2015–19. Despite a growth of 68% in female first and last authorship over a decade, women comprised only 31.8% of first authors and 22.7% of senior authors in the evaluated high-impact journals. Interestingly, the proportion of female first authors was more significant than that of the American Board of Ophthalmology-certified female ophthalmologists in the United States, suggesting that female residents comprise a certain percentage of first authorship in this discipline. While these numbers indicate progress, significant disparities remain here, especially in senior positions. Women ophthalmologists appeared to publish more frequently than expected as first authors relative to their representation in the field, but senior authorship continued to lag.

Pulmonary medicine exhibits similar trends, as highlighted by Geng et al. [13]. The authors conducted a cross-sectional analysis of 12 journals with the highest impact rankings in pulmonary medicine. Female first authors constituted 37%, while last authorship remained at 22%, indicating barriers to leadership roles. From a global perspective, Asia showed the lowest representation of female first (27.6%) and last (15.2%) authors; conversely, Oceania had the highest numbers of female first (46.2%) and last (25.5%) authors. Predictive analysis suggested a parity in female first and last author contributions by 2046 and 2059, respectively. The study also noted that male-authored articles were cited more frequently, while articles with female first and last authors demonstrated the lowest citation counts, opening discussions on systemic bias influencing citation choices and the overall impact of themes and results published. Furthermore, the number of citations significantly affects career prospects in academia, including advancement to full professorships and securing third-party funding.

Contrary to pulmonary medicine, Selvakumar et al. [14] reported much lower numbers of female authorship in a wide range of surgical literature. Studies chosen for meta-analysis included subspecialties such as neurosurgery, orthopedic surgery, plastic surgery, and transplant surgery. The meta-analysis evaluated 15 studies of gender distribution in authorship. The so-called meta-proportion of female first authorship was 20.6% and nearly double that of female last authorship at 11.9%. Compared to the proportion of the female surgical workforce in the United States, which had shown a moderate rise between 2007–19 from 13.6% to 22% in general surgery and 11.9% to 17.2% in plastic surgery, respectively, the total number of female authorship proportion still lags.

The proportion of women in gynecological subjects, on the other hand, presents a more optimistic outlook for the future. Penn et al. [15] examined publications in the leading subspecialty journal, *Gynecologic Oncology*, from its first edition in

1972 through 2014. They discovered a significant increase in female authorship, rising from 11% of female first authors and 0% of female last authors in 1972 to 58% and 37%, respectively, by 2014. Consistent with studies in other medical fields, a female last author was more likely to work with a female first author than her male counterpart (54.2% versus 28.7%). Regarding the composition of the editorial board, women were absent in 1972/73 and 1980, and their representation showed a gradual increase from 3% in 1990 to 9% in 2000. By 2014, 30% of board members were female. A more diverse group of primary decision-makers in a journal can significantly reduce bias and thus contribute to the increasing percentage of publications by women in gynecological oncology.

Rickard et al. [16] examined 750 papers on specific diseases in pediatric urology concerning the academic degree, demographics, and gender parity of the first authors between 1990 and 2019. Only 30% of the coauthors and 21% of the first authors were female when analyzed over the entire period. A predictive analysis showed a continuous increase in female corresponding authors at 55% and female first authors at 83% in 2049. Based primarily on the positive predictive values of the analysis, the authors came to a positive conclusion of increasing participation of female authors in pediatric urology, which is in line with the steadily growing numbers of female specialists in this medical discipline.

Jengahir et al. [17] examined author trends within 30 years between 1987 and 2017 in three major journals focusing on pediatric surgery. They also found a significant increase in female first authorship from 17% in 1987 to 42% in 2017. Within the 30 years, there was also a 19% increase in the total number of authors per journal, which could indicate increasing research participation by clinicians in general and increased competition in academic medicine. As in the study by Rickard et al [16]. described above, the gender shares of senior authorships were not analyzed, which means that the evaluation of the final results lacks an essential factor that, in contrast to the first authorships, is more meaningful concerning the continued academic career of women and their advancement.

Table 3.1 lists an overview of studies published between 2019 and 2023 on gender trends in authorship of different medical disciplines.

Table 3.1 Selected overview of studies published between 2019 and 2023 on gender trends in authorship of different medical disciplines

Author	Year	Journal	Medical disciplines analyzed	Title
Huang et al.	2019	*Cureus*	Radiology	Gender differences in article citation metrics in radiology
Gadek et al.	2023	*Journal of Perinatology*	Neonatology	Gender analysis of authorship during COVID-19
Elias et al.	2023	*J Hosp Med*	General and hospital medicine	Gender differences in COVID-19-related manuscript authorship by hospitalists during the pandemic: a bibliometric analysis

(continued)

Table 3.1 (continued)

Author	Year	Journal	Medical disciplines analyzed	Title
Rubulotta et al.	2022	*Eur J Intern Med*	Internal medicine	Gender distribution in boards of internal medicine societies and paper authorship: networking is the key to success
Beland et al.	2023	*Urology*	Urology	Authorship in urology: a gender reveal
Jagsi et al.	2006	*N Engl J Med*	Internal medicine Obstetrics/ gynecology Pediatrics Surgery	The "gender gap" in authorship of academic medical literature—a 35-year perspective
Yamamura et al.	2023	*BMC Med Educ*	Radiology Urology Surgery Gynecology Pediatrics	Gender differences and cooperation in medical authorships—an analysis of the recent ten years in five key medical disciplines
Hornstein et al.	2022	*JCO Glob Oncol*	Oncology	Authorship equity and gender representation in global oncology publications
Ghattas et al.	2021	*J Bone Joint Surg Am*	Orthopedics	Trends in female authorship in orthopaedic literature from 2002 to 2021: an analysis of 168,451 authors
Fathy et al.	2021	*JAMA Ophthalmol*	Ophtalmology	Female editorial authorship trends in high-impact ophthalmology journals
Geng et al.	2023	*Pulmonology*	Pulmonology	Gender equity of authorship in pulmonary medicine over the past decade
Selvakumar et al.	2023	*Am Surg*	Surgery	Gender distribution and rank of authorship in surgical literature
Penn et al.	2019	*Gynecol Oncol Rep*	Gynecologic oncology	The gender authorship gap in gynecologic oncology research
Rickard et al.[a]	2020	*Urology*	Pediatric urology	Authorship publishing trends and forecasting in pediatric urology: are we closer to gender equality?
Jehangir et al.[a]	2019	*Pediatr Surg Int*	Pediatric surgery	Publishing trends in *Journal of Paediatric Surgery, Pediatric Surgery International* and *European Journal of Pediatric Surgery* over the past three decades

[a]Senior authorship was not analyzed

3.3 Summary

This chapter explores the gender disparities in academic authorship across various medical disciplines, with a particular focus on radiology compared to other fields. While significant progress has been made by women in academic medicine, particularly in research authorship, substantial gaps persist, especially at senior levels. In Radiology, female first authorship increased from 13% in 1984 to 31.5% in 2014, yet senior authorship remains underrepresented. In contrast, disciplines such as pediatrics and obstetrics have seen greater gender balance in research authorship, while fields like surgery and urology continue to demonstrate notable gender imbalances. Various factors contribute to these disparities, including the proportion of female practitioners in each field, structural and networking barriers, societal norms, and biases in citation practices. Notably, subspecialties with higher female physician representation tend to have more gender-balanced research contributions.

The relatively higher gender parity in fields like gynecology and pediatrics can be attributed to several key factors. One of the most important factors is the higher representation of women in the workforce in these fields. With more female practitioners, there is a natural increase in female involvement in research and academic publishing. Another critical factor is the presence of supportive networks and mentorship opportunities, particularly among women. In disciplines like ophthalmology and orthopedics, collaborative networks of female researchers have played a key role in advancing gender equity by supporting the career development of other women in the field.

In addition, disciplines that have made structural changes and become more aware of gender biases have also seen greater gender parity in authorship. Fields such as gynecology have made significant strides by increasing the diversity of editorial boards and leadership teams, which in turn has contributed to a higher representation of women in published research. Furthermore, cultural factors in certain disciplines also play a role. For example, pediatrics benefits from a higher proportion of female practitioners, leading to more balanced gender representation in authorship.

For other medical disciplines, particularly those with lower female representation, adopting these strategies could contribute to greater gender equity in academic publishing. Increasing the number of female practitioners in a field, providing targeted mentorship programs, addressing citation biases, and ensuring more women are placed in leadership roles within research and editorial boards could all foster better gender parity in these fields.

3.4 Conclusion

The examination of gender equality in medical research and authorship reveals significant interdisciplinary differences. While some fields, such as pediatrics, gynecology, and neonatology, have made remarkable strides toward gender parity in first authorship, other disciplines like radiology, surgery, and urology continue to exhibit substantial gender gaps, particularly at senior levels. Persistent systemic barriers, such as the "leaky pipeline" phenomenon and lower citation rates for female-authored work, hinder the advancement of women in academic medicine. The evidence highlights that mentorship programs, institutional support, and targeted interventions are critical for fostering an equitable environment. Disciplines that actively address these issues, such as pediatrics and neonatology, demonstrate that proactive measures can lead to significant progress. However, for fields like radiology and surgery to achieve similar advancements, concerted efforts are needed to address structural barriers, increase visibility for female researchers, and ensure equal opportunities for leadership roles.

References

1. Huang M, Naser-Tavakolian K, Clifton M, Franceschi AM, Kim D, Zhang JZ, Schweitzer M. Gender differences in article citations by authors from American institutions in major radiology journals. Cureus. 2019;11(8):e5313.
2. Gadek L, Dammann C, Savich R, Mmuo-Oji C, Barrera L, Gallagher PG, Machut K. Gender analysis of Journal of Perinatology authorship during COVID-19. J Perinatol. 2023;43(4):518–22.
3. Elias RM, Bonk N, White AT, et al. Gender differences in COVID-19- related manuscript authorship by hospitalists during the pandemic: a bibliometric analysis. J Hosp Med. 2023;18:209–16.
4. Rubulotta F, Santonocito C, Rubulotta G. Gender distribution in boards of internal medicine societies and paper authorship: networking is the key to success. Eur J Intern Med. 2022;97:34–5.
5. Sebo P, Clair C. Gender gap in authorship: a study of 44,000 articles published in 100 high-impact general medical journals. Eur J Intern Med. 2021;97:103. https://doi.org/10.1016/j.ejim.2021.09.013.
6. Beland L, Jeng G, Aibel K, Aro T, Kreshover JE. Authorship in urology: a gender reveal. Urology. 2023;172:224–7.
7. Huen KH, Lee CT, Skinner EC, et al. Women leaders in academic urology: the views of department chairs. Urology. 2020;150:81.
8. Jagsi R, Guancial EA, Worobey CC, Henault LE, Chang Y, Starr R, Tarbell NJ, Hylek EM. The "gender gap" in authorship of academic medical literature – a 35-year perspective. N Engl J Med. 2006;355(3):281–7.
9. Yamamura J, Molwitz I, Ozga AK, Nguyen TA, Wedekind I, Wolf-Baldauf L, Kamo M, Zhao J, Can E, Keller S. Gender differences and cooperation in medical authorships – an analysis of the recent ten years in five key medical disciplines. BMC Med Educ. 2023;23(1):68.
10. Hornstein P, Tuyishime H, Mutebi M, Lasebikan N, Rubagumya F, Fadelu T. Authorship equity and gender representation in global oncology publications. JCO Glob Oncol. 2022;8:e2100369.
11. Ghattas YS, Kyin C, Grise A, Glasser J, Johnson T, Druskovich K, Cannada LK, Service BC. Trends in female authorship in Orthopaedic literature from 2002 to 2021: an analysis of 168,451 authors. J Bone Joint Surg Am. 2023;105(16):1285–94.
12. Fathy CA, Cherkas E, Shields CN, Syed ZA, Haller JA, Zhang QE, Sharpe J, Garg Shukla A. Female editorial authorship trends in high-impact ophthalmology journals. JAMA Ophthalmol. 2021;139(10):1071–8.
13. Geng F, Ren Y, Hou H, Dai B, Scott JB, Strickland SL, Mehta S, Li J. Gender equity of authorship in pulmonary medicine over the past decade. Pulmonology. 2023;29(6):495–504.

14. Selvakumar S, Zagales I, Newsome K, Spardy J, Santos R, Boneva D, Stein DM, Kornblith L, Bilski T, Elkbuli A. Gender distribution & rank of authorship in surgical literature. Am Surg. 2023;89(6):2665–76.
15. Penn CA, Ebott JA, Larach DB, Hesson AM, Waljee JF, Larach MG. The gender authorship gap in gynecologic oncology research. Gynecol Oncol Rep. 2019;29:83–4.
16. Rickard M, Hannick JH, Blais AS, Wang J, Santos JD, Lorenzo AJ. Female authorship publishing trends and forecasting in pediatric urology: are we closer to gender equality? Urology. 2020;139:141–50.
17. Jehangir S, Barnes EH, McDowell D, Holland AJA. Publishing trends in Journal of Paediatric Surgery, Pediatric Surgery International and European Journal of Pediatric Surgery over the past three decades. Pediatr Surg Int. 2019;35(4):413–8.

4 Research and Publications: An International Comparison of Female Representation

Isabel Molwitz, Katharina Ronstedt, and Sarah Keller-Yamamura

4.1 Introduction

Gender parity has not been reached in academic radiology. Despite increasing numbers of female medical students, women remain underrepresented in academic leadership positions. Causes are multifactorial, ranging from individual career aims to structural discrimination, especially concerning family care work. However, the status of gender parity and barriers to overcome vary depending on the region. Measures to ensure equity should be tailored to address cultural and local structural variances.

This chapter provides an overview of the status of gender parity in academic radiology in different regions based on the literature. Potential barriers and effective measures to reach gender parity are discussed.

I. Molwitz
Department of Diagnostic and Interventional Radiology and Nuclear Medicine, University Medical Center Hamburg-Eppendorf (UKE), Hamburg, Germany
e-mail: i.molwitz@uke.de

K. Ronstedt
Department of Pediatric Radiology, Kassel Hospital GmbH, Kassel, Germany
e-mail: Katharina.Ronstedt@gnh.net

S. Keller-Yamamura (✉)
Department of Radiology, Charité-Universitätsmedizin Berlin, Corporate Member of Freie Universität Berlin and Humboldt-Universität zu Berlin, Berlin, Germany
e-mail: sarah.keller@charite.de

S. Keller-Yamamura, J. Yamamura (eds.), *Inclusive Radiology: Fostering Diversity and Equity in Academic and non-Academic Settings*,
https://doi.org/10.1007/978-3-032-05705-1_4

4.2 Gender Parity in Radiological Research in US, European, and Asian Journals

Gender parity in academic radiology varies depending on the region. In an analysis of n = 24,182 publications published between 2007/8 and 2017/18 in European, US, and Asian journals, female authors were underrepresented, especially in Asian journals [1]. In US journals, the number of female first authors increased from 34% to 45% between 2007/8 and 2017/18. Female first authors' representation in European journals increased from 15% to 40%. However, they remained scarce in Asian journals, with 8% in 2007/8 and 13% in 2017/18 [1]. In 2017/18, female first authors were thus more than three times as frequent in radiological US journals than in Asian journals (OR 3.55 [95% confidence interval (95%-CI) 2.62–4.8], $p < 0.0001$). Also, they were significantly better represented in European than in Asian journals (OR 1.49 [95% CI 1.07–2.08], $p = 0.0119$) [1]. These numbers must be compared to the overall number of female radiologists in the corresponding region to assess a potential underrepresentation. This will be addressed later in this chapter.

First authors are usually young academic professionals at the beginning of their careers, while last or senior authors represent research group leaders and advanced academic career positions. As women are less represented in leading positions in radiology, it is not surprising that female last authors are less frequent than female first authors. In the same study, in US journals, their percentage changed from 19% to 24%, in European journals from 9% to 19%, and in Asian journals from 6% to 9% [1].

In 2017/18, female last authors were thus nearly four times as frequent in US than in Asian journals (OR 3.73 [95% CI 2.93–4.75]) and more than twice as frequent in European than in Asian journals (OR 2.78 [95% CI 2.16–3.57]) [1].

Now, what if we look at the number of female radiologists in these regions to assess a potential underrepresentation.

While more than half of medical students in the United States are female [2], women constitute about 35% of all academic radiologists in the United States. The percentage of women depend on the radiological subspecialty, ranging from 12% in interventional radiology to 35% in abdominal imaging, or 45% in pediatric radiology in a 2022 study [3]. Only in breast imaging did women constitute more than half (79%) of all radiologists [3]. Among academic radiologists in the United States, the same study reported 31% female executive-level faculty members, but only 26% female full professors [3]. While female authors in US journals do not necessarily have US affiliations, let us assume this to enable a general assessment. With 45% female first authors in US journals in 2017/18, women would thus be well represented compared to the 35% female academic radiologists. However, women would be underrepresented as last authors in US journals (24%) compared to the 31% of female executive-level faculty members.

Similarly, at least half of all medical students in Europe are female [4]. Female members of the European Society of Radiology make up 30%, among the generation Y 41% [5]. However, only 21% of European chairs in Radiology are held by women [5]. In Germany, about 35% of senior faculty are female [6], but only two chairs and clinical directorships are held by women. The number of female first authors of 40% in European journals thus reflects a good representation of the young generation (generation Y). Female last authors (19%) would be underrepresented compared to senior faculty (at least in Germany).

The investigated Asian journal was Japanese. About 24% of radiologists in Japan are female [7]. Both first (13%) and last female authors (9%) are thus underrepresented compared to the overall number of female radiologists. Another study that evaluated author provenance for articles in the top 50 radiological journals published between 2018 and 2020 during the COVID-19 pandemic found Asian female first authors were more frequent (16%) than North American (10%) or European (9%) [8]. Also, they observed 15% Asian female last authors, 9% North American female last authors, and 5% European female last authors [8]. These findings demonstrate that female authors with Asian affiliations publish more frequently in non-Asian journals [9]. Still, even when comparing 16% female first authors from Asia and 15% female last authors from Asia to the number of female radiologists in, for example, Japan (24%), women from Asia would be underrepresented as leading authors. Compared to female radiologists in Korea (40%) or Thailand (80–90%), underrepresentation of Asian women as first and last authors would be even worse [10].

4.3 Gender Parity in Radiological Research in Australian, African, and Oceanian Journals

In Australia, a clinical radiology workforce census analyzing data from Royal Australian and New Zealand Clinical Radiology found an increase in female radiologists from 13% to 29% between 1992 and 2020 [11]. However, only 13% were chief executives of hospitals with more than 1000 beds (38% of hospitals of all sizes) [12].

For the *Journal of Medical Imaging and Radiation Oncology* from The Royal Australian and New Zealand College of Radiologists, a slight increase of female first authors was observed from 31% in 2012 to 38% in 2020. In the same journal, the number of female last authors increased from 19% in 2012 to 32% in 2020 [13]. Thus, female first authors (38%) were even overrepresented compared to the overall number of female radiologists (29%). Female last authors (32%) were just slightly less frequent than female executives (38%).

Interestingly, in the same journal in 2021 a temporary decrease occurred for female first authors to 28% and for female last authors to 23% [13]. This sharp decrease is likely associated with the COVID-19 pandemic. It has been observed - not only for radiology [8] but across the medical and scientific world [14]- that while overall article numbers increased during the pandemic, female authors were strikingly underrepresented. It is usually hypothesized that this was due to the higher amount of care work that women are traditionally responsible for and which they took on during closed institutional childcare [15, 16].

Concerning Africa and Oceania, a title and abstract search in PubMed, the global standard for biomedical literature [17], for "female authors" AND "radiology"

AND "Africa / Oceania" did not yield any results. This demonstrates an urgent need for more research on this subject, to ensure transparency about gender gaps in academic radiology in these regions. Especially, as, for example, an analysis of the Health Professions Council of South Africa (HPCSA) database of imaging personnel from 2002 to 2019 stated the number of female radiologists increased from 18% to 31% [18]. Also, African radiological journals exist, even though they are of low impact, for example, the *South African Journal of Radiology* (Impact factor (IF) 2023 0.7) or the *West African Journal of Radiology* (IF 2022 < 0.1). Authors are free to submit to journals outside their regions, meaning authors of these journals do not automatically stem from African institutions. However, these journals could lead the debate for Africa by calling for submissions on the topic of gender parity in African journals or analyses of authors with African affiliations in other journals.

One study that asked radiological societies about their numbers of female radiologists, found 35% female radiologists in New Zealand as a part of Oceania [10]. Again, no articles on the representation of female authors from Oceania were found.

In summary, if across all continents, there are increasing numbers of female radiologists and women are region-dependent already well represented as first authors, what is preventing gender parity in other regions and in last author positions?

4.4 Barriers to Gender Parity in Radiological Research Across Regions

Based on interviews with 30 medical leaders in Australia on perceived gender barriers, three aspects were identified: perceptions of capability, capacity, and credibility [12]. "Perception of capability" relates to worse self-esteem of women, including self-doubt, lack of self-confidence, and underestimating personal capabilities [12]. "Capacity" was defined as the incompatibility of career and motherhood with resulting part-time work. This was the most frequently named aspect. Additionally, it was stated that seniors demanded to "just fit in" instead of offering flexible work models [12]. Finally, concerning "credibility", it was noted that women were taken less seriously and that in leadership positions, stereotype male behaviors were demanded regardless of gender [12].

Evidence from other studies supports that women's competence is doubted because they do not fit into the typical leadership image of, for example, a strong and dominant man [19]. However, women cannot simply imitate male leadership behavior. On the opposite, as an article from *Harvard Business Review* states, if women's behavior seems too assertive and masculine, they may be seen as competent but not likable; if their behavior is too feminine, they may be seen as likable but incompetent [20]. Especially, the aspect of family care work is also stressed by many studies. One survey among 76 US radiologists found female respondents to significantly more often report a negative stigma associated with pregnancy than their male colleagues (61% vs. 15%; $p < 0.001$) [21]. Besides a subconscious bias, this might be due to women taking on the family care work. For example, male US radiologists mainly reported not taking a parental leave, while women reported a leave of 10 weeks ($p < 0.001$) [21]. Another study indicates that male radiologists rely on their partners to care for their children [22]. On the contrary, female radiologists are responsible for childcare in their partnerships and consecutively more dependent on institutional childcare [22]. This means that in regions or situations like the COVID-19 pandemic with reduced availability of institutional childcare, women are hindered from pursuing an academic career. The disadvantages of having children seem to be well-known among women. Indeed, a study of 1056 women physicians, mainly from the United States, reported that even though knowing the risks of late motherhood, 76% delayed family plans, and 37% experienced infertility when finally deciding to start a family [23]. Of physicians with children, 47% stated to have passed up on opportunities for career advancement [23]. Nearly five percent (4%) stopped working in medicine entirely [23].

While a positive development concerning female first authors can be observed, there thus seem to be continuous barriers hindering women from reaching senior faculty positions, which is then mirrored by low female last author numbers.

4.5 Potential Measures for Gender Parity in Radiological Research

As the causes are multifactorial, so must be the measures to target gender parity in research. One might differentiate between personal support, organizational support, and cultural aspects.

Personal support would include encouragement from female role models. These women can serve as mentors. Female mentors are especially beneficial as evidence shows that both genders prefer same-sex mentorships [22, 24]. However, successfully building a personal connection [25], mutual respect, shared values, and experience of the mentor are more critical key characteristics of successful mentoring than the mentor's and mentee's gender [26]. As there are only few female senior faculty who can serve as mentors, potential mentees and experienced academic radiologists should consider mentoring independent of their respective gender. Mentors can support the perception of capability and self-esteem of mentees. Apart from mentoring, peers of any gender can nurture women's efforts to establish careers in academic leadership [12]. Mentoring may also help to find a leadership style independent from the male stereotype but still functional for women.

Furthermore essential are organizational aspects, such as implementing flexible work times and transparent appointment processes [12]. Radiology is well suited for adapting new work models such as flexible work times, part-time, or home office. With regard to appointment processes, it is typically stated that "applications from female or disabled/candidates with severe disability (>50%) are welcomed and preferred given an equivalent qualification." It seems a bit ironic to name gender in one phrase with disabilities, thus suggesting female gender to be a disability per se. Independent of the gender debate, it is also questionable to demand that someone disabled should be equivalent to someone who is not disabled. In that case, this person would not be disabled (at least not concerning the job position). Indeed, the overall proportion of radiologists with disabilities is low and further decreases at higher ranks [27]. While a defined qualification level is necessary and should be a promotion prerequisite, transparent application processes could give points to, for example, publications, grant money, years used to care for family members, and potential disabilities. Applicants with the most points could then be chosen if predefined requirements are met.

Concerning professional culture, we should critically reflect our images of the "typical leadership personality" and be aware that we might subconsciously judge women's competency as lower than that of their male colleagues. An innovative approach would be to consider medical careers less linear with fixed promotion ages, which automatically results in disadvantages for women with children, but rather consider promotions to executive and chief positions also at older ages. Why should, for example, people in their fifties who, independent of their gender, took care of their children, ill, or old family members for some years but still managed to achieve a suitable number of publications and grants not be considered for such positions?

4.6 Conclusion

Region-based assessment of gender parity in research is hindered, as most studies evaluate female author representation in specific journals or from journals of a certain region but do not consider the authors' affiliations or origin. Comparisons of regional female author numbers and the number of radiologists from the corresponding journals' region, for example, between authors in US journals and US radiologists, demonstrate a good representation of women as first authors in US and European journals. Female last authors in US and European journals remain underrepresented compared to the proportion of executive-level female radiologists. Compared to the number of Asian female radiologists, women from Asia were underrepresented especially in Asian journals. Data for Australia, Africa, and Oceania is scarce. From available studies, women seem to be well represented as female first authors in Australia and slightly underrepresented as last authors. For Africa and Oceania, data was insufficient to allow valid conclusions. This could be because not only women but radiologists from the entire region are underrepresented in radiological research, and there may be a lack of awareness of gender issues in these regions.

Gender parity in research could be hindered by personal perception of capabilities and low self-esteem of women. More importantly, the competency of female leaders is generally judged less high than that of male leaders. Lacking support of seniors for flexible work times also plays a role. Especially emphasized by many studies are the difficulties of combining academic careers with having children, as women are globally—to different degrees—responsible for family care work and dependent on institutional childcare support. This frequently results in women passing up on career opportunities or not having a family.

Potential measures to target these barriers include mentoring, also by male mentors, peer support, organizational structures such as flexible work models, and application processes that truly represent family care work. Finally, we should rethink our professional culture, a potential subconscious bias toward women in leadership positions, and reflect on alternatives to stringent linear careers with fixed age limits for promotions.

References

1. Molwitz I, Keller S, Wolf-Baldauf L, et al. Female author representation differs between journals from The United States of America, Europe, and Asia: a 10-year comparison of five medical disciplines. Scientometrics. 2023;128:1583–600.
2. Colleges AoAM. Total U.S. MD-Granting Medical School Enrollment by Race/Ethnicity (Alone) and Gender. 2023. Available via https://www.aamc.org/media/6116/download. Accessed 13th January 2025.
3. Goswami AK, Kokabi N, Khaja MS, et al. Academic radiology in the United States: defining gender disparities in faculty leadership and academic rank. Acad Radiol. 2022;29:714–25.
4. Kuhlmann E, Ovseiko PV, Kurmeyer C, et al. Closing the gender leadership gap: a multicentre cross-country comparison of women in management and leadership in academic health centres in the European Union. Hum Resour Health. 2017;15:2.
5. Kubik-Huch RA, Vilgrain V, Krestin GP, et al. Women in radiology: gender diversity is not a metric-it is a tool for excellence. Eur Radiol. 2020;30:1644–52.
6. Ärztinnenbund D. Update: medical women on top. 2022. Available via https://www.aerztinnenbund.de/downloads/8/MWoT2022_Web.pdf. Accessed 10.01.2024.
7. Yamashiro T, Kumamaru KK, Kido A, et al. Work-style reform and use of information and communication technology among diagnostic radiologists in Japan: results of the 2018 JRS/JCR joint survey. Jpn J Radiol. 2020;38:636–42.
8. Quak E, Girault G, Thenint MA, Weyts K, Lequesne J, Lasnon C. Author gender inequality in medical imaging journals and the COVID-19 pandemic. Radiology. 2021;300:E301–7.
9. Molwitz I, Keller S, Wolf-Baldauf L, et al. Female author representation differs between journals from The United States of America, Europe, and Asia: a 10-year comparison of five medical disciplines. Scientometrics. 2022;128:1583–600.
10. Cater SW, Yoon SC, Lowell DA, et al. Bridging the gap: identifying global trends in gender disparity among the radiology physician workforce. Acad Radiol. 2018;25:1052–61.
11. Lim W, Gupta N, Mandel C. Analysis of gender in radiology in Australia and its importance to the profession and workforce planning. J Med Imaging Radiat Oncol. 2023;67:170–8.
12. Bismark M, Morris J, Thomas L, Loh E, Phelps G, Dickinson H. Reasons and remedies for under-representation of women in medical leadership roles: a qualitative study from Australia. BMJ Open. 2015;5:e009384.
13. Batumalai V, Kumar S, Sundaresan P. Trends in gender of first and senior authors of articles published in JMIRO. J Med Imaging Radiat Oncol. 2023;67:179–84.
14. Pinho-Gomes AC, Peters S, Thompson K, et al. Where are the women? Gender inequalities in COVID-19 research authorship. BMJ Glob Health. 2020;5:e002922.
15. Davis PB, Meagher EA, Pomeroy C, et al. Pandemic-related barriers to the success of women in research: a framework for action. Nat Med. 2022;28:436–8.
16. Zamarro G, Prados MJ. Gender differences in couples' division of childcare, work and mental health during COVID-19. Rev Econ Househ. 2021;19:11–40.
17. UC_Merced_Library. Introduction to PubMed. 2024.
18. Mkhize N, Tiwari R, Chikte U, Pitcher R. Temporal trends in the south African diagnostic radiology workforce (2002-2019). Cureus. 2022;14:e27148.

19. Yousaf R, Schmiede R. Barriers to women's representation in academic excellence and positions of power. Asian J Ger Eur Stud. 2017;2:2.
20. Eagly A, Carli LL. Women and the labyrinth of leadership. Harvard Business Review. 2007. Available via https://hbr.org/2007/09/women-and-the-labyrinth-of-leadership. Accessed 26-01 2025.
21. Burkard-Mandel LE, Saadah M, Hahn LR, Wien MA, Hemal U. The impact of the radiology career on family planning: a survey of practicing radiologists and trainees. Clin Imaging. 2024;113:110208.
22. Molwitz I, Kemper C, Stahlmann K, et al. Gender- and personality-specific differences in academic qualifications, research motivation, and attractiveness of leadership positions: a survey among radiologists from Germany. Rofo. 2024; https://doi.org/10.1055/a-2415-7337.
23. Bakkensen JB, Smith KS, Cheung EO, et al. Childbearing, infertility, and career trajectories among women in medicine. JAMA Netw Open. 2023;6:e2326192.
24. Bernard C, Pommier R, Vilgrain V, Ronot M. Gender gap in articles published in European Radiology and CardioVascular and Interventional Radiology: evolution between 2002 and 2016. Eur Radiol. 2020;30:1011–9.
25. Levine RB, Mechaber HF, Reddy ST, Cayea D, Harrison RA. "A good career choice for women" female medical students' mentoring experiences a multi-institutional qualitative study. Acad Med. 2013;88:527–34.
26. Straus SE, Johnson MO, Marquez C, Feldman MD. Characteristics of successful and failed mentoring relationships: a qualitative study across two academic health centers. Acad Med. 2013;88:82–9.
27. Manik R, Sadigh G. Diversity and inclusion in radiology: a necessity for improving the field. Br J Radiol. 2021;94:20210407.

Women's Representation in Current Areas of Healthtech: Artificial Intelligence

5

Lisa Adams

5.1 Introduction

Artificial intelligence (AI) has rapidly become a cornerstone of innovation in healthcare, particularly in radiology and other imaging-heavy fields. Many analysts regard AI-driven computer vision algorithms as a catalyst for more accurate and efficient disease detection, for enabling diagnostic support in under-resourced settings, and for propelling the transformation of clinical decision-making. While enthusiasm about the potential of AI continues to mount, there is also increasing recognition that these technologies can inadvertently reinforce long-standing inequities if not developed and deployed conscientiously. Sex- and gender-based disparities, in particular, risk being amplified by data-driven processes that treat entire populations as homogeneous or neglect the distinct biological and societal factors that shape healthcare experiences for women.

The underrepresentation of women in AI affects outcomes in at least two distinct ways. First, there is underrepresentation of women as subjects within training datasets, which can limit the ability of algorithms to perform accurately for female patients. Second, there is underrepresentation of women in research and leadership roles, an imbalance that decreases the likelihood of identifying and rectifying blind spots in the AI development pipeline. Without deliberate action on who is included in the data and who develops the systems, AI can underdiagnose or misclassify conditions in female patients. Researchers in biomedical informatics, medical imaging, and ethics have increasingly underscored the significance of these issues, although much work remains to be done to implement solutions at scale [1, 2].

L. Adams (✉)
Institute of Diagnostic and Interventional Radiology, School of Medicine and Health, University Hospital of Technical University Munich, Munich, Germany
e-mail: lisa.adams@tum.de

S. Keller-Yamamura, J. Yamamura (eds.), *Inclusive Radiology: Fostering Diversity and Equity in Academic and non-Academic Settings*,
https://doi.org/10.1007/978-3-032-05705-1_5

AI, however, is not inherently destined to perpetuate inequalities. Well-designed algorithms, curated with a representative distribution of patients across biological sexes and gender categories, can reveal diagnostic patterns that are especially relevant to women's health. Such designs have the potential to reduce disparities by identifying subtle imaging findings that might be overlooked in traditional workflows. They can also help increase awareness of sex- and gender-based differences in disease pathophysiology, supporting more personalized treatment plans. The critical question is how radiologists, data scientists, healthcare institutions, and policymakers can collaborate to shape AI systems that promote equity rather than exacerbate historical gaps.

5.2 The Development of AI-Based Tools in Radiology and Healthtech

Advances in computational methods have fueled the incorporation of AI into radiology. Machine learning algorithms, including deep neural networks, are capable of parsing complex imaging data to detect lesions, classify disease phenotypes, and generate risk scores for individual patients [3]. In principle, these capabilities could reduce the workload of radiologists, who face expanding imaging volumes in many parts of the world. As triage and prioritization support, AI can highlight suspicious areas in scans or flag cases that warrant urgent attention, potentially improving both the speed and accuracy of diagnosis [4]. Through the integration of additional patient data—such as laboratory findings, genomic profiles, and even social determinants of health—AI further aspires to support nuanced clinical decisions.

Early milestones in AI for medical imaging centered on simpler machine learning classifiers or rule-based expert systems, but the introduction of deep convolutional neural networks advanced the field substantially. When trained on large datasets, these networks excel at tasks including automated segmentation of anatomical regions, detection of microcalcifications in mammography, and characterization of lung nodules in chest CT scans [5]. However, the success of such networks depends largely on the robustness and comprehensiveness of the training data. If training samples neglect certain subpopulations-or deviate from real-world sex and gender distributions, algorithmic performance can deteriorate for the underrepresented groups. That deterioration might go unnoticed if developers and regulatory agencies fail to scrutinize performance metrics by subgroup, an oversight that invites misdiagnoses in clinical settings.

A separate, though equally consequential, challenge emerges from the complexity of biological sex and social gender constructs, particularly in clinical contexts as present for example in cardiology, oncology, and endocrinology. Certain diseases present differently in women, sometimes with distinct or subtler imaging findings, and these nuances can escape an AI model that was never trained on an adequate sample of female cases [6, 7]. Additionally, social factors that disproportionately affect women, such as delayed access to medical care or increased exposure to caregiving responsibilities, can shape the clinical scenario in which scans are taken and the stage at which disease is detected. AI models that use aggregated variables may fail to capture these layered realities, further marginalizing women in diagnostic processes.

Crucially, the development pipeline for AI in radiology has rarely mandated sex-specific or gender-specific analyses. Many software developers focus on maximizing overall performance—measured through metrics like accuracy, sensitivity, or specificity aggregated across the entire dataset—without differentiating subgroups. This can hide the fact that high overall accuracy might be driven largely by strong performance in the majority class, often male patients in many datasets. Explainability does not substitute for subgroup auditing. Report stratified performance and calibration by sex and evaluate errors by subgroup [8].

5.3 Data Imbalances and Consequences for Female Patients

One of the most critical issues in AI-driven healthcare is the well-documented imbalance in medical imaging datasets. Large repositories like CheXpert [9] have become standard benchmarks. However, it was previously indicated that male patients can be overrepresented in some of these datasets, depending on the institution from which the images originate and the medical conditions for which patients were referred [10]. This phenomenon may partially reflect the prevalence of specific diseases among men, but it can also stem from structural biases in healthcare access or from the fact that certain health complaints more commonly prompt men to undergo imaging. In cardiology, for instance, men historically receive more diagnostic imaging referrals for chest pain than women, often due to the mistaken belief that cardiovascular disease primarily affects men [11, 12]. Over time, such referral patterns distort the representation of men and women in datasets, resulting in an algorithm that "learns" from a skewed sampling of patients. If an AI model is fine-tuned to detect abnormalities based on predominantly male-type presentations of disease, it may fail to recognize the subtler or atypical presentations more common among women, thus widening the gap in timely and accurate diagnosis.

These disparities can translate into systematic errors. An algorithm might exhibit robust performance in classifying pneumonia or identifying cardiomegaly on chest X-rays for male patients but falter when analyzing the same diseases in women, especially if the latter population was less prevalent during training [1]. The mismatch between the training data distribution and real-world demographics is a fundamental source of algorithmic bias. Although rebalancing techniques—such as oversampling, undersampling, or employing specialized loss functions—offer partial remedies, they depend on first acknowledging the imbalance and adjusting data handling accordingly. Institutions may need to invest considerable effort into collecting additional imaging data from underrepresented groups to ensure that algorithms are both fair and generalizable.

A closely related point concerns the labeling of sex and gender within these datasets. Many imaging repositories do not distinguish "sex" (the biological attribute) from "gender" (the social or identity-based attribute), and some do not systematically record either. Lack of consistent demographic annotation makes it difficult to separate performance outcomes by subgroup. Even advanced performance analyses may only classify patients as "male" or "female" without delineating factors such as hormone levels, pregnancy status, or other clinical details that bear on disease manifestation [13]. This coarseness obscures significant within-group variation among female patients. Additionally, algorithms often ignore social gender roles, cultural contexts, or socioeconomic determinants that influence disease progression and healthcare access. Although addressing these aspects is more complex than balancing raw sex-based data, it is necessary to ensure that AI systems are truly representative and equitable in practice.

5.4 Hidden Pathways of Bias in the AI Pipeline

Bias in AI for radiology is not confined to data collection alone but rather can emerge at multiple stages in the pipeline [14]. During data annotation, for instance, if the labeling team lacks detailed guidelines on how certain pathologies might present differently in men and women, they might uniformly label specific radiographic findings without tagging relevant sex-specific markers. Annotation protocols that fail to differentiate the presence of reproductive organs, hormone-related changes, or postpartum status can obscure relevant patterns. This oversight is particularly concerning for conditions like breast cancer, where subtle factors such as breast density and microcalcification distribution may be critical to detection [15].

Model selection also exerts an influence on how biases manifest. Neural network architectures are known for their high capacity to detect patterns, but they do not inherently identify whether those patterns are valid across subpopulations. If the hyperparameter tuning is oriented only toward maximizing aggregate metrics such as overall accuracy, there is no built-in mechanism to prevent worse performance on female patients [16]. Techniques like fairness-aware machine learning, reweighting, or adjusting class weights can mitigate some of these concerns, yet they remain uncommon in mainstream medical AI research. Furthermore, evaluating performance across subgroups requires additional computational resources and more detailed analysis, something that many time-pressed research groups or product teams may not prioritize.

After model development, validation processes can further conceal inequities if test datasets are similarly unbalanced or if evaluation metrics are not stratified by sex. External validation on data from geographically distinct institutions is recommended to ensure that the model generalizes beyond the training environment, but sex-specific sub-analyses are often not mandatory. Even if institutions track overall sensitivity, specificity, and area under the ROC curve (AUC), these measures can disguise large differences across subpopulations. Researchers may be satisfied with a robust average performance, inadvertently obscuring the fact that female patients experience lower-quality results [17]. Once deployed, AI tools can generate feedback loops that reinforce existing biases. If the model under-diagnoses certain conditions in women, those cases may not be flagged for follow-up imaging or additional interventions, leading to fewer data points from that subgroup being collected in the future [18]. Over time, this cyclical effect can codify a partial or incomplete understanding of disease expression in female populations, making subsequent AI systems even less representative. Although human-in-the-loop structures could catch such discrepancies, they hinge on radiologists and clinicians actively monitoring how the algorithm performs across demographics, which is not guaranteed if departmental resources are already stretched thin.

5.5 Underrepresentation of Women in AI Leadership and Research

When discussing sex and gender disparities in healthtech, it is vital to consider that these issues extend beyond the nature of the data itself. The composition of research and development teams significantly influences whether biases are identified, prioritized, and corrected. Women remain markedly underrepresented in senior roles within radiology, computer science, and AI-driven research, creating an environment in which decisions are disproportionately shaped by male viewpoints [19, 20]. At academic conferences devoted to machine learning and AI, female participation as speakers or primary authors often lags behind men. This shortfall is further accentuated at the leadership level, where men predominate on editorial boards, conference committees, and grant review panels. When relatively few women hold decisive roles, it becomes less likely that resource allocation, publication opportunities, and strategic priorities will systematically address gaps affecting female patient populations [21].

In many clinical departments, including radiology, a smaller proportion of women achieve full professorship, chair positions, or directorships compared to men, partly due to institutional cultures and societal expectations around caregiving responsibilities. These barriers restrict the diversity of perspectives that shape what kinds of AI tools get funded, what research questions are deemed important, and which stakeholder partnerships are pursued. If primarily male-led teams develop AI solutions, they may focus on conditions and data sources that reflect their own clinical experiences, inadvertently sidelining diseases that more frequently or uniquely affect women.

Mentorship, sponsorship, and role modeling are also critical. Junior female scientists often look for experienced mentors who can guide them in translating their technical skills and research interests into grant proposals, publications, and leadership roles. If few senior women exist in AI-driven fields, the mentorship capacity for the next generation is limited, perpetuating a cycle in which talented women move to other areas or encounter persistent glass ceilings [22].

Addressing the imbalance requires structural and cultural efforts. Institutional policies that promote work–life balance, fair compensation, and transparent evaluation criteria for promotion can help retain female professionals in AI and radiology. Funding bodies can also implement measures to encourage diversity among principal investigators and within research consortia, thereby expanding the variety of viewpoints that guide data governance and algorithmic design. Professional societies, including the Radiological Society of North America (RSNA) and the European Society of Radiology (ESR), have begun to intensify their focus on equity, but practical, measurable changes are necessary for these initiatives to be effective over the long term (WiML, n.d., *Our Mission*, https://wimlworkshop.org/; Women in Global Health, n.d., *Gender Equity Hub*, https://womeningh.org).

5.6 Strategies for Addressing Sex- and Gender-Based Disparities in AI

Multiple approaches can mitigate the risk of perpetuating or amplifying sex- and gender-based disparities in AI-driven medicine. One prominent suggestion is to enforce more rigorous standards for dataset documentation. Journals, conference organizers, and regulatory bodies could require researchers to report the sex and gender composition of their training and test sets. This practice would enable peer reviewers, clinicians, and patients to see explicitly whether AI performance was evaluated across demographic subgroups. Authors could be asked to provide metrics such as sensitivity, specificity, or area under the ROC curve separately for men, women, and potentially other self-reported gender identities or relevant subgroups [23, 24].

External validation, already seen as a cornerstone of robust AI development, should incorporate datasets that approximate diverse real-world settings. This diversity includes geographic, racial, ethnic, and sex-based representation. A model that performs exceedingly well in a single hospital with a skewed population may not generalize to broader contexts. By sharing aggregated results by sex, developers can detect if underperformance occurs for certain subgroups and work on rebalancing or redesigning the algorithm before deployment [25]. Institutions can tackle the problem of unbalanced datasets by investing resources in targeted data collection efforts. If an institution recognizes that its cardiac imaging dataset predominantly features men, it can recruit more women to ensure sex parity, possibly through dedicated outreach or collaborations with specialized clinics. Additional imaging data from conditions that predominantly affect women—for instance, fibroids or endometriosis—can also expand the scope of training sets, yielding a more comprehensive picture of female health. A partial solution is the use of data augmentation and synthetic data generation, though real-world data is typically preferred for its fidelity to clinical complexity and variability.

Fairness-aware machine learning techniques offer another line of defense. Tools such as reweighting, adversarial debiasing, and group-aware loss functions aim to ensure that performance remains consistent across predefined demographic categories [26]. While such methods are more commonly discussed in the context of racial and socioeconomic disparities, there is a growing literature on incorporating sex- and gender-related constraints into the training process. Integration of these techniques can penalize models that disproportionately misclassify female cases, effectively nudging the solution toward a more equitable balance.

Promoting the representation of women in radiology and AI leadership can have a profound impact. Funding agencies and professional societies can award grants specifically designed to support female-led AI research. Institutions can develop mentorship programs that match junior female radiologists or data scientists with more seasoned female investigators who have successfully navigated academia or industry leadership. Networking organizations, such as WiML, have demonstrated the effectiveness of community-building in increasing women's visibility at major conferences and supporting collaborative research initiatives. Through such sustained efforts, more women will acquire the resources and opportunities needed to shape cutting-edge AI projects, influencing everything from data collection practices to the interpretation of model outputs.

Ethical oversight and transparency are equally critical. Institutional Review Boards (IRBs) can mandate explicit explanations of how sex and gender considerations are handled in AI research protocols. Journals can echo this stance, asking authors to articulate what steps they took to prevent sex-based or gender-based biases, how they collected and labeled data, and how they evaluated subgroup performance. Such a shift in the publication culture can incentivize more rigorous study designs. A number of leading health journals support that authors disaggregate results by sex for clinical trials, and extending these policies to AI-based diagnostic tools is a logical next step [23, 27].

5.7 Opportunities for AI to Improve Women's Health

Although concerns about bias loom large, there is substantial optimism that AI can also be a force for progress in women's health. In mammography, deep learning models can detect early-stage breast cancer, including microcalcifications or subtle masses that humans might overlook, thereby reducing both false negatives and false positives [15]. When algorithms are trained on well-curated and demographically balanced datasets, they show promise in refining risk stratification, recommending personalized screening intervals, and flagging suspicious findings that might require additional imaging or biopsy.

Outside of breast imaging, AI can enhance the detection of gynecological conditions such as ovarian cysts or uterine fibroids if data is collected systematically from female patients. Research also suggests that advanced algorithms can assist in prenatal imaging, helping to diagnose fetal anomalies with greater precision [28, 29]. In each of these instances, the model's success relies on robust datasets that accurately reflect the female physiology and clinical context, as well as on interdisciplinary teams that include both imaging experts and specialists in women's health.

In cardiology, many institutions are beginning to account for sex-based differences in myocardial perfusion [30], plaque composition, and vessel diameter when using AI to interpret cardiac MRIs or CT angiography scans. With enough training data reflecting female pathophysiology, algorithms can learn to pick up early markers of ischemic heart disease that might manifest differently in women compared to men. Such personalization could lead to earlier diagnoses and more nuanced management protocols, especially if combined with risk factors like hormone profiles, pregnancy history, or autoimmune conditions more prevalent in women.

Moreover, AI's capacity to integrate social determinants of health with clinical data is another avenue for addressing disparities. If algorithms can incorporate variables like socioeconomic status, geographic access to healthcare facilities, or caregiving burdens—factors that frequently disadvantage women in healthcare systems—they may serve as an alert mechanism for high-risk, underserved patients [2]. Rather than ignoring these complexities, a well-structured AI pipeline can highlight the need for more proactive interventions, thereby diminishing gaps in care for vulnerable women.

5.8 Looking Forward: Reconciling Innovation with Equity

The impact of AI on disparities depends on whether developers, clinicians, funders, and regulators embed equity requirements from the outset. Pre-specify sex-disaggregated reporting, stratified calibration, subgroup error analysis, and decision-curve evaluation, and make deployment contingent on meeting predefined equity targets.

Cultural changes within academia, industry, and medicine must parallel these technical actions. Departments can strive to recruit more women faculty with expertise in data science, possibly through cluster hires or targeted fellowships. Partnerships with organizations like Women in Machine Learning or Women in Global Health can connect medical institutions to broader networks of female AI professionals, enriching research agendas and ensuring knowledge exchange. Such initiatives may also improve the retention of women in the workforce as they see clear opportunities for professional advancement, collaboration, and leadership.

Professional societies have begun issuing policy statements on AI ethics, some of which address bias mitigation, though many remain at an abstract level. Converting these statements into robust guidelines that detail operational steps—for instance, specifying the percentage of female representation required in any reference dataset—would bridge the gap from concept to practice. Similarly, journals and funding agencies that champion open-science practices can encourage the release of annotated datasets containing key demographic variables and sex labels, helping other researchers replicate or extend fairness-oriented approaches [31].

When AI is developed and validated with an awareness of demographic diversity, it can better capture the full range of human physiology and disease manifestations. For women in particular, this approach can rectify historical neglect in certain research domains and deliver clinically meaningful gains, whether through enhanced early detection of breast cancer, more accurate cardiac diagnostics, or personalized screening schedules. Equitable AI thus holds the promise of a more inclusive era of precision medicine, in which each patient's unique biological and social context is a foundational element of clinical decision-making.

References

1. Larrazabal AJ, Nieto N, Peterson V, Milone DH, Ferrante E. Gender imbalance in medical imaging datasets produces biased classifiers for computer-aided diagnosis. Proc Natl Acad Sci. 2020;117(23):12592–4.
2. Obermeyer Z, Powers B, Vogeli C, Mullainathan S. Dissecting racial bias in an algorithm used to manage the health of populations. Science. 2019;366(6464):447–53.
3. He K, Zhang X, Ren S, Sun J. Deep residual learning for image recognition. In: Proceedings of the IEEE conference on computer vision and pattern recognition; 2016. p. 770–8.
4. Hosny A, Parmar C, Quackenbush J, Schwartz LH, Aerts HJ. Artificial intelligence in radiology. Nat Rev Cancer. 2018;18(8):500–10.
5. Kermany DS, Goldbaum M, Cai W, et al. Identifying medical diagnoses and treatable diseases by image-based deep learning. Cell. 2018;172(5):1122–31. e1129
6. Regitz-Zagrosek V. Why do we need gender medicine? Sex and gender aspects in clinical medicine. Springer; 2011. p. 1–4.
7. Regitz-Zagrosek V. Therapeutic implications of the gender-specific aspects of cardiovascular disease. Nat Rev Drug Discov. 2006;5(5):425–39.
8. Chen JH, Asch SM. Machine learning and prediction in medicine—beyond the peak of inflated expectations. N Engl J Med. 2017;376(26):2507.
9. Irvin J, Rajpurkar P, Ko M, et al. Chexpert: a large chest radiograph dataset with uncertainty labels and expert comparison. In: Proceedings of the AAAI conference on artificial intelligence; 2019. p. 590–7.
10. Paul HY, Kim TK, Siegel E, Yahyavi-Firouz-Abadi N. Demographic reporting in publicly available chest radiograph data sets: opportunities for mitigating sex and racial disparities in deep learning models. J Am Coll Radiol. 2022;19(1):192–200.
11. Ravn-Fischer A, Karlsson T, Santos M, Bergman B, Herlitz J, Johanson P. Inequalities in the early treatment of women and men with acute chest pain? Am J Emerg Med. 2012;30(8):1515–21.
12. Bösner S, Haasenritter J, Hani MA, et al. Gender bias revisited: new insights on the differential management of chest pain. BMC Fam Pract. 2011;12:1–8.
13. Krieger N. Genders, sexes, and health: what are the connections—and why does it matter? Int J Epidemiol. 2003;32(4):652–7.
14. Glocker B, Jones C, Roschewitz M, Winzeck S. Risk of bias in chest radiography deep learning foundation models. Radiology. Artif Intell. 2023;5(6):e230060.
15. Yala A, Lehman C, Schuster T, Portnoi T, Barzilay R. A deep learning mammography-based model for improved breast cancer risk prediction. Radiology. 2019;292(1):60–6.
16. Hardt M, Price E, Srebro N. Equality of opportunity in supervised learning. Adv Neural Inf Proces Syst. 2016;29.
17. Adamson AS, Smith A. Machine learning and health care disparities in dermatology. JAMA Dermatol. 2018;154(11):1247–8.
18. Aikens RC, Chen JH, Baiocchi M, Simard JF. Feedback loop failure modes in medical diagnosis: how biases can emerge and be reinforced. Med Decis Mak. 2024;44:0272989X241248612.
19. Yan TD, Yuan PH, Saha T, Lebel K, Spalluto L, Yong-Hing CJ. Female authorship trends among articles about artificial intelligence in North American radiology journals. Can Assoc Radiol J. 2023;74(2):264–71.
20. Busch F, Keller S, Rueger C, et al. Mapping gender and geographic diversity in artificial intelligence research: editor representation in leading computer science journals. Acta Radiol Open. 2023;12(10):20584601231213740.
21. Edwards JB, Tudiver F. Women's preventive screening in rural health clinics. Womens Health Issues. 2008;18(3):155–66.
22. Silver JK. Six practical strategies to mentor and sponsor women in academic medicine. J Med Internet Res. 2023;25:e47799.
23. Clayton JA, Tannenbaum C. Reporting sex, gender, or both in clinical research? JAMA. 2016;316(18):1863–4.

24. Chung H, Park C, Kang WS, Lee J. Gender bias in artificial intelligence: severity prediction at an early stage of COVID-19. Front Physiol. 2021;12:778720.
25. Yang Y, Zhang H, Gichoya JW, Katabi D, Ghassemi M. The limits of fair medical imaging AI in real-world generalization. Nat Med. 2024;30(10):2838–48.
26. Dwork C, Hardt M, Pitassi T, Reingold O, Zemel R. Fairness through awareness. In: Proceedings of the 3rd innovations in theoretical computer science conference; 2012. p. 214–26.
27. Granton D, Rodrigues M, Raparelli V, et al. Sex and gender-based analysis and diversity metric reporting in acute care trials published in high-impact journals: a systematic review. BMJ Open. 2024;14(5):e081118.
28. Moradi B, Taherian R, Tahmasebpour AR, et al. Fetal corpus callosum abnormalities: ultrasound and magnetic resonance imaging role. J Clin Ultrasound. 2022;50(7):989–1003.
29. Ramirez Zegarra R, Ghi T. Use of artificial intelligence and deep learning in fetal ultrasound imaging. Ultrasound Obstet Gynecol. 2023;62(2):185–94.
30. Hachamovitch R, Berman DS, Kiat H, et al. Effective risk stratification using exercise myocardial perfusion SPECT in women: gender-related differences in prognostic nuclear testing. J Am Coll Cardiol. 1996;28(1):34–44.
31. Arora A, Alderman JE, Palmer J, et al. The value of standards for health datasets in artificial intelligence-based applications. Nat Med. 2023;29(11):2929–38.

Part II

Barriers and Facilitators to Career Advancement

Career Prospects in Clinical Radiology, Areas of Interest, and Barriers to Advancement

6

Sarah Keller-Yamamura and Isabel Molwitz

6.1 Introduction

Clinical radiology represents a dynamic and evolving field at the intersection of technology and medicine. With the growing demand for imaging services, advancements in diagnostic modalities, and expanding subspecialties, radiology offers a plethora of career opportunities. However, the path to professional and academic advancement in radiology is often riddled with challenges. This chapter explores career prospects in clinical radiology, highlights areas of interest, and discusses barriers to advancement with a particular focus on the German healthcare context. Furthermore, it synthesizes findings from recent surveys and research, including gender-specific and structural factors influencing career trajectories.

6.2 The Scope of Clinical Radiology

Radiology is integral to modern medicine, encompassing diagnostic, interventional, and therapeutic roles. Key subspecialties include neuroradiology, musculoskeletal imaging, pediatric radiology, breast imaging, and interventional radiology. Beyond clinical roles, radiologists contribute significantly to medical education and research,

S. Keller-Yamamura (✉)
Department of Radiology, Charité-Universitätsmedizin Berlin, Corporate Member of Freie Universität Berlin and Humboldt-Universität zu Berlin, Berlin, Germany
e-mail: sarah.keller@charite.de

I. Molwitz
Department of Diagnostic and Interventional Radiology and Nuclear Medicine, University Medical Center Hamburg-Eppendorf (UKE), Hamburg, Germany
e-mail: i.molwitz@uke.de

S. Keller-Yamamura, J. Yamamura (eds.), *Inclusive Radiology: Fostering Diversity and Equity in Academic and non-Academic Settings*,
https://doi.org/10.1007/978-3-032-05705-1_6

with opportunities to explore artificial intelligence applications, molecular imaging, and precision diagnostics.

6.3 Academic Careers in Radiology

Academic radiology provides a platform for combining clinical practice with research and teaching. In Germany, the pathway to an academic career requires formal qualifications, including obtaining the "Habilitation," a postdoctoral qualification necessary for becoming a professor. The Habilitation process involves significant research contributions, publications in high-impact journals, and successful teaching evaluations. Mentorship plays a critical role, with structured mentoring programs helping candidates navigate these requirements.

Statistics indicate that globally, women are underrepresented in academic radiology leadership. For example, out of 34.7% female academic radiologists in the United States, 30.6% reach the executive level [1]. In Germany, only 15% of female academic radiologists are department heads at medical faculties [2] compared to significantly higher percentages of their male counterparts. This disparity is attributed to structural barriers, including limited mentorship opportunities, uneven distribution of research funding, and work–life balance challenges.

Beyond the Habilitation, academic advancement also depends on obtaining competitive grants, building collaborations, and achieving high citation metrics. Protected research time is a crucial factor, with institutions providing varying levels of support to academics. German radiologists have expressed satisfaction with existing protected research time; however, funding disparities remain a hurdle for many, particularly women [3, 4]. Studies also suggest that women in academic radiology are promoted slower than men and stagnate particularly in the middle career stages [5]. The reasons are multifactorial and range from personal preferences to infrastructural weaknesses, little support from mostly male superiors and pronounced marginalization [6, 7]. Other studies have shown that female doctors in academia spend more time teaching and advocating, which is less relevant for career promotion in Germany than in Anglo-American culture. Leadership in radiology also involves contributing to national and international committees, peer-reviewed journal boards, and professional societies. Despite efforts to increase female representation, women often face challenges in these areas due to implicit biases and fewer sponsorship opportunities [8, 9]. Addressing these disparities requires systemic reforms and targeted diversity initiatives.

6.4 Impact of the COVID-19 Pandemic

The COVID-19 pandemic has amplified existing disparities in academic medicine. It disproportionately affected women's career advancement and research output, particularly for those with caregiving responsibilities. Studies have shown a marked decline in research productivity among women in academia during the pandemic.

The increased burden of childcare and homeschooling, combined with clinical demands, left many female academics with reduced time for scholarly activities. Female radiologists reported fewer publications and grant submissions compared to their male counterparts during this period [10, 11].

Women with young children faced the most significant challenges, with surveys indicating higher levels of burnout and job dissatisfaction. This has raised concerns about long-term impacts on career trajectories, including delayed promotions and reduced representation in leadership roles [12, 13]. Institutions must address these inequities by implementing flexible work policies, providing targeted support for caregivers, and fostering an inclusive environment to ensure the retention and advancement of talented female academics. With a little imagination for a more future-oriented career promotion of women and caring parents, a kind of points system for the achievement of academic milestones would also be conceivable, so that women and men could receive points for caring for children, for example, during parental leave and maternity leave, in order to compensate for stagnating research performance to a small extent and thus maintain gender competition and parity in the allocation of management and research positions.

6.5 International Trends

Globally, radiology is witnessing increasing demand for professionals adept in cutting-edge technologies such as machine learning and genomics. Career prospects are bolstered by collaborative opportunities across borders, facilitated by organizations such as the European Society of Radiology and the Radiological Society of North America. However, gender disparities persist in leadership roles across countries. For instance, in the United States, women comprise approximately 20% of full professors in radiology, and only about 10–15% hold department chair positions. These numbers reflect slow progress despite various diversity initiatives [9, 14]. In Japan, women are significantly underrepresented in radiology leadership positions. A 2022 study highlighted that only 4.7% of professors across various academic fields in Japan are women, indicating a steep decline in female representation at higher academic ranks [15]. In the broader medical community, women physicians are vastly underrepresented in the leadership structures of Japanese professional medical societies [16]. This underrepresentation is part of a wider societal issue in Japan, where women occupy a small fraction of leadership roles across various sectors. For instance, the Japanese government has set a target for women to hold at least 30% of executive positions in private companies by 2030, acknowledging the current disparity [17]. Efforts are ongoing to address these disparities and promote gender equality in leadership positions within radiology and other fields in Japan. While German radiology mirrors US numbers, with 13% of heads of medical faculties, the percentage of women in leadership positions is lower [2]. A study focusing on academic interventional radiologists found that only 18% of chief physicians and 22% of senior physicians were women in Germany [18]. In general radiology, where the proportion of women has increased over time, they still hold a marginal role in top and leading positions [19]. Efforts are ongoing to address these disparities and promote gender equality in radiology leadership in Germany. In Italy, women are underrepresented in radiology leadership, holding only 11.2% of full professor positions, 31.6% of associate professors, and 34.7% of researcher roles. Despite almost equal numbers of women choosing radiology as a career in Italy, there is a significant gender gap at senior academic levels, with only 14% of heads of radiology departments being women [20]. Contributing factors include systemic barriers in academia and healthcare institutions, leading to slow progress toward gender equality in leadership positions.

These different national examples highlight the critical role of cultural and systemic factors in shaping gender representation in radiology leadership. Countries with supportive policies, such as childcare support and flexible work arrangements, tend to have higher percentages of women in leadership roles. Conversely, nations with traditional gender norms and insufficient structural support like Japan seem to face more pronounced disparities.

6.6 Potential of New Areas of Interest in Radiology

The increasing complexity of medical care has driven growth in radiological subspecialties. Areas such as molecular imaging, interventional oncology, and hybrid imaging modalities (e.g., PET/MRI) are gaining prominence. Radiologists specializing in these fields often find opportunities in academia and industry, contributing to innovation and clinical trials. These areas can be particularly suitable for radiologists with care work responsibilities. Many subspecialties allow for predictable schedules and less on-call duty compared to general or interventional radiology. The highly focused nature of these subspecialties often supports a balanced workload and provides opportunities for part-time or flexible employment arrangements. Also, artificial intelligence (AI) is revolutionizing radiology by enhancing diagnostic accuracy, optimizing workflows, and improving efficiency. Radiologists with expertise in AI and informatics are at the forefront of this transformation, opening new career pathways in research, development, and technology leadership. Careers in AI and informatics often involve roles in academia or industry that prioritize project-based work, making them well-suited for radiologists seeking flexibility to accommodate family duties. Remote work possibilities and collaboration through digital platforms further enhance work–life balance for professionals in this field.

Radiology's role in personalized medicine is expanding, with imaging biomarkers aiding in tailored therapeutic strategies. Radiologists who engage in research involving biomarkers and theranostics are highly sought after in academia and industry. The emphasis on research and development in personalized medicine often provides structured schedules and the possibility of remote collaboration, aligning well with the needs of radiologists managing family commitments.

Teleradiology is another area of radiology that is increasingly attractive for professionals with family responsibilities. It allows radiologists to interpret images and provide diagnostic reports remotely, offering a high degree of flexibility in work hours and location. This adaptability is particularly beneficial for parents or caregivers, enabling them to manage clinical responsibilities alongside personal obligations. Teleradiology also supports international collaboration, providing access to diverse clinical cases while maintaining a flexible working arrangement.

Radiologists pursuing careers in industry have diverse pathways, including roles in medical imaging companies, pharmaceutical firms, and healthcare technology startups. These professionals contribute to the development of imaging equipment, software solutions, and AI-powered diagnostic tools, driving innovation in radiology practice. They may work as product managers, clinical researchers, data scientists, or consultants, focusing on improving diagnostic accuracy and workflow efficiency. Careers in industry often offer flexibility, including opportunities in regulatory affairs, marketing, and sales, allowing radiologists to blend clinical expertise with technology and economic leadership. The increasing demand for radiologists in industry-driven roles ensures growth in both academia and commercial sectors, contributing to advancements in imaging and personalized medicine.

6.7 Barriers to Advancement in Radiology

As already described in the upper sections, a vast majority of studies published in recent years highlight that despite the increasing number of female radiologists globally, women remain underrepresented in leadership roles. In Germany, male radiologists are four times more likely to have acquired an associate professorship (Habilitation Privatdozent) compared to their female counterparts [3]. Furthermore, men are more likely to plan and achieve such qualifications, underscoring a significant disparity. Mentorship plays a pivotal role in addressing these gaps, with female mentees often preferring female mentors, although their availability is limited [3, 4].

To enhance the attractiveness of leadership positions, female radiologists emphasize the importance of gender balance at the management level, top sharing, and better work–life balance [3, 4]. These measures, combined with systemic changes in mentorship and sponsorship programs, are essential to fostering equity in academic advancement.

Mentorship plays a pivotal role in career development, particularly in academic medicine. It provides guidance, support, and opportunities for learning that are crucial for career progression [21]. Mentorship helps mentees build networks, enhance their professional skills, and gain insights into navigating complex institutional landscapes. In the German medical system, mentorship structures are influenced by historical, institutional, and cultural factors. The proportion of female radiologists in senior positions is still relatively low, limiting the availability of female mentors for junior female radiologists. This imbalance results in unequal access to same-sex mentorship opportunities, for women in male-dominated fields such as radiology.

A study on mentorship in academic radiology found that male radiologists tend to receive more mentorship support, particularly when it comes to advancing academic qualifications (like publishing, grant applications, and career progression) [22]. Female radiologists, on the other hand, often prefer female mentors as they may find shared experiences and perspectives beneficial. However, their opportunities to connect with senior female mentors are limited due to the smaller pool of women in senior academic roles [23, 24].

Balancing clinical responsibilities with academic pursuits and personal life is a significant challenge. Surveys indicate that better work–life balance, including flexible schedules, part-time opportunities, remote work options, and top-sharing positions, are key to making leadership positions more attractive, particularly for women [3, 4, 25]. Employers in clinical radiology can significantly enhance work–life balance by implementing several strategies: *Flexible scheduling:* Offering flexible hours or compressed workweeks allows radiologists to balance clinical duties with personal responsibilities. Additionally, job sharing, allowing two professionals to share a full-time role, can enable continuity of care while supporting individual flexibility. For example, in the United Kingdom, several radiology departments have implemented successful job-sharing arrangements, where two part-time radiologists collaborate on cases, ensuring consistent patient care while accommodating personal schedules. *Childcare support:* Providing on-site childcare facilities or childcare services subsidies can alleviate working parents' stress. For instance, Scandinavian countries such as Norway and Sweden provide state-subsidized childcare options and parental leave policies that have significantly increased workforce participation among radiologists with young children. Parental leave in these countries is among the most generous in the world. In Sweden, parents are entitled to 480 days of paid leave per child, which can be shared between both parents. Norway offers 49 weeks of fully paid leave or 59 weeks at 80% pay, with a portion reserved specifically for fathers to encourage shared caregiving responsibilities [26]. Additionally, as of July 1, 2024, Sweden introduced a policy allowing parents to transfer up to 45 days of their parental leave to grandparents or other close family members. This initiative aims to provide families with greater flexibility and support during the early stages of a child's life [27]. Germany offers a relatively comprehensive parental leave system. Parents are entitled to up to 36 months of parental leave, which can be divided between them as they choose until the child reaches the age of eight. Additionally, "Elterngeld" (parental allowance) provides income replacement for up to 14 months, with 2 months reserved for the nonprimary caregiver to promote equitable caregiving [28]. Japan provides up to 12 months of paid parental leave at approximately 67% of salary for the first 6 months and 50% for the remaining period. However, cultural norms often dissuade fathers from taking leave, and working mothers may face challenges in returning to their careers due to traditional expectations and limited childcare support [29]. France offers 16 weeks of fully paid maternity leave for the first child, increasing to 26 weeks for the third child. Fathers are entitled to 28 days of paternity leave, which includes 7 days of compulsory leave. France also provides subsidized childcare options, including crèches and allowances, to support working parents [30]. In contrast, the United States has no federally mandated paid parental leave, leaving most working parents dependent on employer-specific policies. As a result, many radiologists in the United States return to work sooner than their counterparts in Nordic or European countries, often within a few weeks of childbirth, which can contribute to higher stress levels and reduced job satisfaction. While some institutions in the United States offer progressive leave policies, these remain exceptions rather than the norm. *Dual-career networks:* Germany's dual-career networks are an integrated support system aimed at helping couples where both partners pursue demanding careers [31]. These networks recognize that achieving a satisfactory balance between professional ambitions and family life is essential—not only for personal well-being but also for retaining top talent. To that end, many institutions and companies offer comprehensive services that go well beyond standard HR practices. For example, specialized offices at universities and large organizations assist the non-academic or nonlocal partner with job searches and career counseling, ensuring that both individuals can find suitable opportunities when relocating for work. In addition, these networks provide tailored relocation support, helping families navigate administrative challenges and integrate into their new communities. Flexible work arrangements—such as part-time opportunities, remote work options, flexible schedules, and even top-sharing positions—are strongly promoted within these frameworks, making leadership roles more accessible and attractive, particularly for women. This holistic approach not only enhances work–life balance but also contributes to greater gender equality in senior and decision-making positions. According to the report "Karrierebündnis Familie und Beruf – Erfolgsfaktoren für die Vereinbarkeit von Familie und Beruf" by the German Federal Ministry for Family Affairs, Senior Citizens, Women and Youth, such initiatives have played a pivotal role in supporting dual-career couples and improving overall job satisfaction in Germany. *Remote work options:* Remote work opportunities, particularly through telemedicine and teleradiology, offer a transformative approach to work–life balance in clinical radiology. Hospitals and imaging centers can establish robust digital infrastructure to enable remote image analysis, reporting, and consultations. For example, combining Picture Archiving and Communication Systems (PACS) and secure virtual platforms allows radiologists to access and interpret imaging studies from home. Remote work reduces commuting time, provides flexibility in managing work hours, and creates opportunities for radiologists to practice across multiple geographic regions. In Canada, for instance, teleradiology networks have been particularly effective in servicing rural areas while enabling radiologists to maintain flexible schedules. Remote options also enhance job satisfaction and retention by accommodating personal and family commitments [32]. Opponents of remote work point out that the advantages of remote work are offset by possible disadvantages, such as the blurring of the boundaries between private and professional life and the fact that employees become available outside regular working hours. However, encouraging policies that foster clear boundaries, such as the prevention of after-hours work communication, can help professionals disengage and recharge effectively. By adopting these measures, institutions can foster an environment that supports radiologists' personal and professional growth while ensuring they remain motivated and productive. The combination of institutional support, cultural shifts, and innovative work models can significantly enhance radiologists' work–life balance and career satisfaction.

6.8 Summarized Strategies for Overcoming Barriers

Enhancing mentorship programs: To mitigate the mentorship gap, institutions should implement structured mentorship programs that include cross-gender mentoring. Encouraging senior male radiologists to mentor female colleagues can help bridge the divide while expanding opportunities for young professionals. In the United States, programs such as the American Association for Women Radiologists' mentorship initiative have successfully increased female participation in academic radiology [33]. These programs focus on connecting early-career professionals with experienced mentors who provide guidance on publishing, grant writing, and career advancement. *Promoting work–life integration:* Flexible work schedules, top sharing, and improved childcare support are essential to fostering work–life integration. Scandinavian countries like Sweden and Norway have demonstrated the effectiveness of providing extensive parental leave, which encourages equitable caregiving roles and allows both men and women to remain engaged in their careers. Similarly, Germany's dual-career networks support academic couples, helping radiologists navigate family commitments without sacrificing professional growth. *Addressing systemic inequalities:* Institutional policies must address systemic biases in recruitment, promotion, and resource allocation. For example, transparent criteria for academic advancement and equitable distribution of research opportunities can help level the playing field. In Australia, initiatives like the Women in Leadership Development Program have focused on creating clear pathways for advancement, leading to a significant increase in female participation in medical leadership roles over the last decade [34]. *Encouraging diversity in leadership:* Achieving gender balance in leadership positions requires proactive measures such as targeted leadership training for women and diversity quotas. Visible female role models can inspire the next generation of radiologists [8]. Countries like Canada have successfully implemented diversity quotas for leadership positions in healthcare, ensuring that hiring committees prioritize gender and cultural diversity. *Leveraging technology:* AI and digital platforms can streamline administrative tasks, allowing radiologists to allocate more time to research and professional development. Institutions should invest in these technologies to support academic productivity. In the United Kingdom, AI tools are increasingly used in radiology departments to handle routine image analyses, freeing up time for radiologists to focus on complex cases and academic pursuits. These innovations can be complemented with virtual collaboration platforms to enhance teamwork across geographical boundaries.

References

1. Sharma S, Malik A, Matschek J, Zaki-Metias KM, Gandhi R, Yong-Hing CJ, Khosa F. Assessing and improving women representation in radiology leadership positions. Curr Probl Diagn Radiol. 2025;54(1):4–10. https://doi.org/10.1067/j.cpradiol.2024.10.021. Epub 2024 Nov 26.
2. DeutscherÄrztinnenbund. Update: Medical women on top. Dokumentation des Anteils von Frauen in Führungspositionen in klinischen FÄchern der deutschen UniversitÄtsmedizin.

2022. Accessed 23 Dec 2024 at: https://www.aerztinnenbund.de/downloads/8/MWoT2022_Web.pdf.

3. Molwitz I, Kemper C, Stahlmann K, Yamamura J, Adam G, Langenbach MC, Reim M, Wegner F, Bannas P, Lotz J, Can E, Zagrosek-Regitz V, Hamm B, Keller-Yamamura S. Gender- and personality-specific differences in academic qualifications, research motivation, and attractiveness of leadership positions: a survey among radiologists from Germany. Rofo. 2024. English, German. https://doi.org/10.1055/a-2415-7337. Epub ahead of print.
4. Molwitz I, Kemper C, Stahlmann K, Oechtering TH, Sieren MM, Afat S, Gerwing M, Bucher AM, Storz C, Langenbach MC, Reim M, Lotz J, Zagrosek-Regitz V, Can E, Köhler D, Yamamura J, Adam G, Hamm B, Keller S. Work expectations, their fulfillment, and exhaustion among radiologists of all career levels: what can be learned from the example of Germany. Eur Radiol. 2023;33(8):5664–74. https://doi.org/10.1007/s00330-023-09510-6.
5. Tesch BJ, Wood HM, Helwig AL, Nattinger AB. Promotion of women physicians in academic medicine. Glass ceiling or sticky floor? JAMA. 1995;273(13):1022–5. https://doi.org/10.1001/jama.273.13.1022.
6. Clark RA. Promotion and retention of women physicians in academia. J La State Med Soc. 2008;160(5):289–91.
7. Levinson W, Tolle SW, Lewis C. Women in Academic Medicine. N Engl J Med. 1989;321(22):1511–7. https://doi.org/10.1056/nejm198911303212205.
8. Magliano DJ, Macefield VG, Ellis TM, Calkin AC. Addressing gender equity in senior leadership roles in translational science. ACS Pharmacol Transl Sci. 2020;3(4):773–9. https://doi.org/10.1021/acsptsci.0c00056.
9. Goswami AK, Kokabi N, Khaja MS, et al. Academic Radiology in the United States: defining gender disparities in faculty leadership and academic rank. Acad Radiol. 2022;29(5):714–25.
10. Vincent-Lamarre P, Sugimoto CR, Larivière V. The decline of women's research production during the coronavirus pandemic. Nature Index. 2020;19.
11. Lee KGL, Mennerat A, Lukas D, Dugdale HL, Culina A. The effect of the COVID-19 pandemic on the gender gap in research productivity within academia. elife. 2023;12:e85427. https://doi.org/10.7554/eLife.85427.
12. Sarma S, Usmani S. COVID-19 and Physician Mothers. Acad Med. 2021;96(2):e12–3. https://doi.org/10.1097/ACM.0000000000003851.
13. Gao J, Yin Y, Myers KR, et al. Potentially long-lasting effects of the pandemic on scientists. Nat Commun. 2021;12:6188. https://doi.org/10.1038/s41467-021-26428-z.
14. Radiological Society of North America (RSNA). A Check-Up on the Progress of Women in Academic Radiology. WIA Report, August 24, 2022. Accessed 27 Dec 2024 at: https://www.wiareport.com/2022/08/a-check-up-on-the-progress-of-women-in-academic-radiology/
15. Nagano N, Watari T, Tamaki Y, Onigata K. Japan's academic barriers to gender equality as seen in a comparison of public and private medical schools: a cross-sectional study. Womens Health Rep (New Rochelle). 2022;3(1):115–23. https://doi.org/10.1089/whr.2021.0095.
16. Watari T, Gupta A, Kataoka H. Representation of gender and postgraduate experience among Professional Medical Society Boards in Japan. JAMA Netw Open. 2022;5(12):e2247548. https://doi.org/10.1001/jamanetworkopen.2022.47548.
17. Asao K, Khera P, Vasishth M. Why such few women in leadership positions in Japan?: Japan. Selected Issues Papers. 2024;2024(024):A001. Retrieved Dec 27, 2024, from https://doi.org/10.5089/9798400281655.018.A001.
18. Blum SFU, Dewald CLA, Becker L, Staudacher E, Franke M, Katoh M, Hoffmann RT, Rohde S, Paprottka PM, Wacker F, Westphalen K, Bruners P, Gebauer B, Das M, Uller W. The status of academic interventional radiologists in Germany with focus on gender disparity: how can we do better? CVIR Endovasc. 2024;7(1):47. https://doi.org/10.1186/s42155-024-00456-4.
19. Fichera G, Busch IM, Rimondini M, Motta R, Giraudo C. Is empowerment of female radiologists still needed? Findings of a systematic review. Int J Environ Res Public Health. 2021;18(4):1542. https://doi.org/10.3390/ijerph18041542.
20. Vernuccio F, Crimì F, Pepe A, Quaia E. Women in radiology: perceived or true barrier? Tomography. 2022;8(4):1881–4. https://doi.org/10.3390/tomography8040158.

21. Fagan RJ, Eskildsen D, Catanzano T, Stanietzky R, Kamel S, Elsayes KM. Burnout and the role of mentorship for radiology trainees and early career radiologists. Diagn Interv Radiol. 2024;30(5):313–7. https://doi.org/10.4274/dir.2024.242825.
22. Bredella MA, Fessell D, Thrall JH. Mentorship in academic radiology: why it matters. Insights Imaging. 2019;10:107. https://doi.org/10.1186/s13244-019-0799-2.
23. Molwitz I, Yamamura J, Ozga AK, Wedekind I, Nguyen TA, Wolf L, Kamo M, Zhao J, Can E, Keller S. Gender trends in authorships and publication impact in Academic Radiology-a 10-year perspective. Eur Radiol. 2021;31(12):8887–96. https://doi.org/10.1007/s00330-021-07928-4. Epub 2021 May 19.
24. Yamamura J, Molwitz I, Ozga AK, Nguyen TA, Wedekind I, Wolf-Baldauf L, Kamo M, Zhao J, Can E, Keller S. Gender differences and cooperation in medical authorships – an analysis of the recent ten years in five key medical disciplines. BMC Med Educ. 2023;23(1):68. https://doi.org/10.1186/s12909-023-04041-6.
25. PraktischArzt. Immer noch eine Aufgabe—Gleichstellung von Ärztinnen (6/7/2020). Available at: https://www.praktischarzt.de/magazin/immer-noch-eine-aufgabe-gleichstellung-bei-aerztinnen/ (assessed 24/02/2025).
26. Swedish Institute 2004. Work–life balance: Sweden has made it easier to combine career with family life. Here's how. Accessed 17 Dec 2024 at https://sweden.se/work-business/working-in-sweden/work-life-balance.
27. Anne-Françoise Hivert. Sweden allows grandparents to take parental leave. Le Monde 2024. Accessed 17 Dec 2024 at https://www.lemonde.fr/en/economy/article/2024/07/06/sweden-allows-grandparents-to-take-parental-leave_6676873_19.html.
28. Handbook Germany. Parental Leave ("Elternzeit"), updated Feb 1, 2024. Accessed 17 Dec 2024 at https://handbookgermany.de/en/parental-leave.
29. Japan Dev. All About Childcare Leave: Paternity and Maternity Leave in Japan. Updated Oct 28, 2023. Accessed 17 Dec 2024 at https://japan-dev.com/blog/paternity-maternity-leave-japan.
30. Oyster. A guide to maternity and paternity leave in France. Published Nov 28, 2024. Accessed 27 Dec 2024 at https://www.oysterhr.com/library/parental-leave-in-france.
31. German Federal Ministry for Family Affairs, Senior Citizens, Women and Youth (BMFSFJ). Karrierebündnis Familie und Beruf – Erfolgsfaktoren für die Vereinbarkeit von Familie und Beruf. 2015. Accessed 24 Feb 2025 at https://www.bmfsfj.de/bmfsfj/themen/familie.
32. Kamineni S, et al. Teleradiology: enhancing access to radiological services in rural areas. J Telemed Telecare. 2005;11(2):82–6.
33. US Department of Labor. Family and Medical Leave (FMLA). Accessed 27 Dec 2024 at https://www.dol.gov/general/topic/benefits-leave/fmla.
34. Sam Hunt. Push for more women in medical leadership this International Women's Day. Med J Aust. 2024;220(4):1. Published online: March 8, 2024. Accessed 27 Dec 2024 at https://www.mja.com.au/journal/2024/220/4/push-more-women-medical-leadership-international-womens-day.

7 Female Mentoring Programs and Their Importance for Career Prospects

Martha Dohna and Kerstin Westphalen

7.1 Introduction

Mentoring is considered one of the key factors for an academic career. Nowadays it is rare to find an organization or institution without a written statement of commitment to diversity, and each year billions of dollars are invested in boosting the representation of women and minorities [1]. Mentoring programs are widespread and have become an integral part of human resources development strategies. Open questions remain in how we define the term mentoring, what types of mentoring programs exist, what influence do medical-academic networks have and how do they affect the success of the mentee? And do mentoring programs contribute to retaining women in academic radiology and are they successful in bringing more women into leadership positions? In this chapter, we wish to explore these questions.

7.2 My Personal Career Story: Was This Mentoring?

As a young radiologist, I made the experience in my hospital that I was not only taught difficult tasks and techniques, but I was also trusted to apply them being passionate about my job. My head physician at the time encouraged me and let me carry out interventions very early on, first guided by him, later alone. He also stood

M. Dohna
Clinic for Diagnostic and Interventional Radiology, University Hospital Bonn, Bonn, Germany
e-mail: Martha.dohna@ukbonn.de

K. Westphalen (✉)
Department of Diagnostic and Interventional Radiology, Evangelical Hospital Hubertus, Berlin, Germany
e-mail: Kerstin.Westphalen@jsd.de

S. Keller-Yamamura, J. Yamamura (eds.), *Inclusive Radiology: Fostering Diversity and Equity in Academic and non-Academic Settings*,
https://doi.org/10.1007/978-3-032-05705-1_7

by my side during lectures as back-up. Retrospectively, I would consider this an informal and not outspoken mentoring relationship. But although he valued my expertise and passed on his knowledge to me, he would nevertheless give the coveted jobs to my male colleagues, as though this was a naturally given rule. For my male colleagues, he would use his power to create job opportunities, better pay, and increasing power. Although we, the female doctors, bore the brunt of the work in the department, we had no say in the development of the department and were not involved in important decisions. We were merely kept informed. Promoting the career and not only the skills of a talented woman seems not to even have occurred to my head physician.

After several years of being omitted again and again for promotion in this department, I accepted the call to another hospital to become head of the department of radiology. For over 14 years now, I built up a large interventional department. And I actively ensure that women in my department not only receive coaching and further training but are offered real career prospects. As president of the 103rd German Radiology Congress in 2022, I put a clear focus on diversity and the promotion of women stating as motto "Living diversity—shaping the future." Today, I would add: "Creating opportunities."

Unfortunately, my personal experience is representative of many female mentees. While men are more often supported by mentors from the senior executive level, women are more likely to be supported by mentors from lower management levels. Female mentees tend to be coached, whereas male mentees are actively supported. Their mentors stand up for their (male) mentees, ensure that the young talents are visible, are considered for promising opportunities, and thus advance their careers. They even negotiate interesting jobs, promotions, and salary increases [2]. Still today, progress in women in leadership positions is frustratingly slow. Two out of 36 (5.6%) university hospital radiology departments in Germany are run by a woman despite 64.6% of female medical students [3]. A large variety of female mentoring programs have been introduced to tackle this gender gap in radiology in Germany.

7.3 Defining Mentoring

To understand the origin of the term mentoring, we need to look back 3300 years to the Trojan War. The historical roots of the term are found in Homer's epos "Odyssey": when Odysseus went to war, he asked his friend Mentor to assure his son's upbringing. The first mentoring program in world history was born [4]. More recent definitions extend this notion: "Mentoring is a relatively stable dyadic relationship over time between an experienced mentor and his or her less experienced mentee. It is characterized by mutual trust and goodwill, and its aim is to promote learning and development as well as the mentee's progress." [5] In other words, mentoring programs aim at providing long-term support and encouragement for the mentee; they are not short-term in nature like coaching but are to function like tandem bike riding where both parties cycle together, and both arrive as joint achievement. They are intended to thoroughly and sustainably serve career development and, ideally, help the mentee achieve a better, higher professional position with the support of the mentor.

7.4 Mentoring Program Designs

Mentoring programs can be organized in very different ways. In one-to-one mentoring, the mentee and mentor enter an exclusive tandem relationship. In group mentoring, several mentees work together with one mentor. In peer mentoring, advice and support are provided by peers within the mentee group. Most university hospitals in Germany and all federal states offer mentoring programs for early career researchers [Mentoring programs for early career researchers—Deutscher Bildungsserver], such as Forum Mentoring, Leibniz Mentoring, or the Talenta career program for women at Frauenhofer.

7.5 Success Outcomes of Mentoring Programs

Mentoring programs have existed in Germany for more than 20 years. The goals of mentoring programs can either focus on the mentee's personal improvement tailored to strengths, passion, wishes, and weaknesses of the mentee, or they can take a more general approach aiming to improve teaching skills and knowledge in areas that are not taught in medical school and are not part of regular professional training. Ideally, mentoring combines both and leads to greater (measurable) overall success for the mentee.

Data evaluating the success and effectiveness of mentoring programs in medicine are rather chastening. The comprehensive systematic review by Sambunjak et al. published in 2006 found no evidence for the effectiveness of mentoring interventions in reducing gender inequalities [6]. 15 years later, in 2021, House et al. conducted a systematic review of the literature and again found no evidence for the effectiveness of mentoring programs in terms of gender equality for female academics in medicine [7]. As a result, they stated that no study provided clear evidence for the implementation of mentoring programs at an institutional level, rather than informally between individuals, as a means of addressing gender inequalities in academic medicine [7].

7.6 Evaluating Success and Effectiveness of Mentoring Programs

In the literature, a major obstacle to the evaluation of mentoring programs appears to be the considerable variability and lack of specificity of the stated aims of different mentoring approaches, of the structures and processes subsumed under the term mentoring, and of the expected or measured outcomes of mentoring programs [7].

The stated goals of mentoring programs and thus the evaluation criteria for the success of mentoring are mostly general statements such as the participants' experiences of academic life and the extent to which they believe it has been positively changed by mentoring. Outcomes are often self-reported and include the participant's experience of better work-life balance, job-related well-being and job satisfaction, general satisfaction, increased self-confidence and self-efficacy, job-related anxiety versus satisfaction, development of networking skills, and better time management [7]. A range of broader, self-reported outcomes can be assessed, such as improved clinical leadership skills, an enhanced national or international profile, pursuing the career path taken and remaining in academic life, and feeling welcomed as a member of the scientific or clinical community [7].

These are important personal outcomes, but they do not assess if mentoring has improved the gender gap in female leadership in medicine for which mentoring programs have initially been introduced.

A larger Australian study [8] on the impact of mentoring programs on women's careers in health and medical research included a list of objectives, for example, knowledge and skills to be more inclusive, understanding of diversity and inclusion, ability to have difficult conversations in the workplace, supervision and team management, personal communication style, professional collaboration, how to chair a meeting, and promotion opportunities. This study shows an interesting design including "knowledge and skills to be more inclusive" and "understanding of diversity and inclusion" as outcome measures for the mentee. This implies that the mentee is seen as a future leader who herself needs to understand inclusion and diversity in order to spread the idea within the institution. Through the study design, the mentee who was exposed to gender inequality became an active agent against gender inequality in the future within the organization. Interestingly, in this study, the mentor was also involved in change and personal progress according to the values of the mentoring program [8].

Despite this well-designed study, overall methodological quality of the studies was moderate to low, making it difficult to determine the program elements most important for success [9]. In summary, although some promising studies with well-defined outcome measures could be found, the success outcomes and educational content of mentoring programs are mostly poorly defined and lack measurable outcomes such as salary increases, higher positions, academic productivity as measured by publications and scholarship income.

7.7 Effects of Mentoring

Although mentoring relationships have been identified as valuable for career advancement, particularly for minority groups, and have been widely integrated into gender equality activities [1, 9], few could be formally evaluated and there is some, but limited, evidence of their effectiveness beyond the immediate satisfaction of participants [8]. But valuable is not synonymous with effective or successful. However, in a systematic review, 10 out of 18 studies reported improvement in representation, promotion, retention, and remuneration [9]. Clear definitions of outcome measures are crucial to evaluate mentoring initiatives whether they achieve their intended goals and whether they justify the human and financial resources invested in them.

The results of Grisso et al. [10] are promising as they found a greater decrease in working hours together with significantly more publications in the group of supervised female PhD students, possibly reflecting a learning effect in terms of "working smarter." However, this result was only found for female faculty with PhDs who are involved in teaching and academics, but not for female doctors with PhDs but not involved in teaching or research, suggesting that interventions should be more intensive or tailored to specific groups of faculties [10].

In the Australian study mentioned above, all mentees were mid-career women, while a third of the mentors were men in top positions. Success was evaluated 12 months after completion of the mentoring program and measured as changes in participants' knowledge, skills, behaviors, and research metrics required for an academic career. The program had a positive impact on receiving scholarships, awards, and other leadership opportunities, as well as resilience. 48% of mentees stated a positive change in promotion opportunities, 30% better grant opportunities, and 26% improved job opportunities [8]. An increase in self-confidence as well as support from their mentors and the network built through the program were seen by participants as essential to achieving these outcomes [8]. The mentees and mentors who participated in the study reported that participation not only improved their personal understanding of the barriers faced by women in healthcare and medical research careers as well as the concepts of diversity and inclusion, but also the skills they can use to be more inclusive in their workplace [8]. This is a crucial finding as change is only possible if men, who hold the majority of positions of power, are included and understand the need for change.

7.8 Initiatives to Reduce Gender Inequality Can Even Have Ironic Consequences: Beware of the "Illusion of Fairness"!

Kaiser et al. [11] showed that the mere presence of diversity structures in a company leads members of high-status groups (white men) to assume that members of underrepresented groups (women) are treated more fairly in that company, regardless of whether the company treats underrepresented groups in the same way as high-status groups. This was despite concrete evidence that women were discriminated, for example, by unjustifiably lower salaries. This "illusion of fairness" resulted in majority group members being less sensitive to recognizing discrimination against minorities and reacting more negatively to minority group members who claimed discrimination [11]. This data suggests that organizations that disregard their diversity policies may convince others and themselves that discrimination claims against them are unfounded, even though there is no evidence that their diversity policies are effective. In an institution that offers an equal opportunity program, creating the "illusion of fairness" could lead to the paradox that those who claim to have experienced discrimination are less likely to be believed. One conclusion from this work is therefore that organizations need to be aware of and actively pay attention to the "illusion of fairness" [11].

7.9 The Problem of Leadership Style: The Struggle with Expectations as a Woman

Women in leadership positions struggle with the expectations placed on them because they are a woman, while at the same time trying to fulfill the expectations of a leader. If they behave like a woman who is quiet, gentle, kind, and loving, they are not perceived as a strong leader. If the female leader behaves in a way that is expected of a leader, namely aggressive, ambitious, dominant, self-confident, and assertive, she will find herself in conflict with not behaving like a woman. In the latter case, she is likely to face rejection and may feel denigrated. In this clash of expectations, people assume that such highly effective women must not be very likeable or nice. Men don't like them, and neither do women. And unfortunately, women do care. We want to please and we want to be popular.

As human expectations are not easily changed, change of workplace settings to reduce gender perception should become an integral part of female mentoring. Female quotas might be a solution to tackle contradicting expectations toward female leaders by avoiding to have a single female member on a team. Not only are women less likely to be overheard by their outnumbered male colleagues, but, especially when they are numerous, they are not assigned the stereotypical roles of "seductress," "mother," "pet," or "iron maiden." This will free women to a certain extent from having to behave in a feminine way as the group can then set a new standard. When women are not just a small minority, their identity as a woman becomes less important and colleagues are more likely to respond to them based on their individual competencies. Ensuring a critical mass of women in leadership positions—not just the one female seat at the table—is an active measure against tokenism female leaders often face [12]. This is a strong argument for female quotas.

Here is some good news: leadership scholar James MacGregor Burns has introduced a leadership framework that distinguishes between transformational and transactional leadership. Transformational leaders act as role models, and gaining the trust of their followers is essential. They are innovative, advise, and empower their subordinates and encourage them. Transactional leaders create give-and-take relationships that appeal to the self-interest of subordinates, correcting and possibly punishing them. Men sometimes adopt a laissez-faire leadership style that takes little responsibility for management. Today, most leaders use a combination of these two leadership styles. Women tend to adopt a more transformational style that encourages other colleagues and subordinates, which is better suited for leading modern organizations. Eagli and Carli conclude that the women's approach is generally more effective, while the men's approach is often less effective or even hinders effectiveness [12].

Many leaders might not have experienced other leadership styles and might therefore be convinced of a transactional leadership style as the gold standard of quality leadership. Now, female leadership style being transformational is genuinely different. But we hopefully all agree that evidence-based data proving female leadership styles to be more successful in modern institutions might show female leadership styles to be different from male leadership styles, but they are as a fact still more successful. To consider this different approach not simply as different but as a lack of quality is merely defending prevalent leadership styles despite data that prove otherwise. Therefore, it is time to critically rethink leadership styles and question prevalent role models.

These results encourage not only to bring more women into leadership positions but also to motivate women to dare to adopt different leadership styles. Rather than talking about mentoring programs and their direct impact on single women, female mentoring programs should be considered under economic aspects as an investment into future sustainability and success of an institution.

7.10 When Women Make Another Women Trip

In general, women have the image of helping each other out and being community oriented. But there are a few exceptions. This is when women deliberately trip other women at work. The behavior, called pink on pink aggression (POPA), consists of a woman with higher power status degrading, ridiculing, or undermining the work of a woman with less power. Such behavior may hinder the career goals of junior female doctors. It is important to understand that POPA is not a conflict of two clashing characters but a unilateral aggression of the more powerful woman toward the woman in the less powerful position. Therefore, mediation and conflict resolution are likely not to be successful as the precondition for successful mediation is that both parties wish to resolve the conflict, and this is not given in POPA. In POPA, the aim of the woman in power is to damage the career of the younger or less powerful woman.

POPA can involve many aspects and actions. To name a few: The older woman in charge of the schedule might consistently give the younger woman a worse schedule including overwhelming and too much work, telling her that she needs to be nicer to the men in the department. The older woman might refuse to teach a particular imaging technique to a younger woman diminishing her in front of the (male) leader. Gossiping and slagging is commonly used by the older woman to diminish the younger woman's entrepreneurial spirit and innovation and undermine her status within the department. The older woman might tell the younger woman that the reasons why she received the job in the department is because she was pretty [13].

Gokli et al. [14] found in a survey carried out among pediatric radiologists in 2022 that of all respondents, nearly half (47%) experienced POPA, while 68% had witnessed such behavior. They also found that 36% of respondents admitted to exerting this behavior on other women. The team reported that while most respondents agreed that such behavior is limited to a few people, 39% ranked pink-on-pink aggression as a middle or top cause of job-related stress and tension. Additionally, 46% indicated that it had changed or affected their career path. Jealousy is reported as top cause for POPA from the female perspective [14].

These numbers show that POPA is unfortunately a widespread phenomenon with possible negative career impact. Therefore, mentoring programs should include both how to deal with POPA but also teach clear behavioral conduct for women to assure that the next leadership generation discontinues this devastating behavior of women competing, comparing, and diminishing each other [15].

7.11 Who Should Be a Mentor? And Why a Sponsor?

Especially in a one-to-one mentoring relationship, both mentor and mentee should be comfortable with each other, feel trust and respect for each other, and should be convinced of the other's skills and abilities. A mutual connection should be present. Both should take time to consider and must have the courage to step out of politeness and comfort into daring honesty to reject a mentoring relationship if one of these preconditions for a fruitful relationship is not given.

Mentees must be respectful with the mentor's time and not passively expect input from the mentor but come prepared, ask questions, and know what help precisely she needs to reach her goal. The mentee must treat the mentor's precious relations he or she is willing to share with the necessary respect and must never overstep. Boundaries set by the mentor must be respected.

A genuine interest in the mentee and matching skills to help are important for the mentor. The mentor should offer *supportive* advice instead of *direct* advice, thus leaving freedom to the mentee to make her own decisions with the information given. "Being a mentor is about asking smart questions, not having all the answers" [16]. The mentor should be willing to speak up for the mentee and should ideally be prepared to be more than a mentor. A mentor offers tailored advice, a sponsor has power, and is willing to use it for his or her mentee. If a mentor is willing to use his or her power and seat at the decision table to create real career opportunities for the mentee, he or she becomes a sponsor willing to be a representative of the mentee, their agent, and committed advocate. A mentor is a nice-to-have, but real career opportunities will not come without a sponsor. A sponsor needs to have a seat at the decision-making table, must have exposure to the mentee's work to have credibility, and needs to have power to achieve the career step for his or her mentee [Carla Harris].

7.12 Keys to Successful Mentoring of Women

The term glass ceiling is widely used and was propagated by former Secretary of State Madeleine Albright, who wears a brooch with a *broken* glass ceiling. This term, coined by Carol Hymowitz and Timothy Schellhardt in the *Wall Street Journal* in 1986, describes an invisible barrier to women's careers in the upper echelons. However, it seems that it is not the ceiling at the end of the road to the top, but the many small setbacks and discriminations throughout their careers that cause this thorough setback for women in leadership positions. The lack of female leaders in companies is the sum of the discrimination that has taken place at all levels, not evidence of any particular barrier to women's progression to the top. Hence, the problem is not the glass ceiling [12]. Mentoring programs must be designed to bring about a general change in attitude and acceptance and to promote an understanding of diversity and inclusion among all members of the institution. Building women's confidence and professional skills is important but can only be successful if it is accompanied by overall change and the will to change from the top. Therefore, all people and especially male leaders should be involved in women's mentoring as they still hold the power today. And only if we can create more understanding of gender discrimination among those in power can real change take place.

For measurable success, it is in most cases important to have sponsorship in addition to mentorship. A mentor will share his or her tailored knowledge with the mentee whereas a sponsor has power and is willing to use it for the mentee. Commonly, successful men have received informal one-to-one mentoring and sponsorship that often transforms into a personal ambition of the mentor/sponsor to demonstrate his power by pushing their mentee to the most possible success. Including those who hold the power as mentors in female mentoring provides the opportunity of sponsorship for the female mentee. Combining sponsorship with mentoring is essential for true success.

7.13 Discussion

Despite numerous mentoring programs for women in medicine, success and effectiveness of such programs are limited and only given if certain criteria of program design are fulfilled. The aim of bringing more women into leadership positions is not sufficiently reached and progress is too slow. Measurable outcomes such as salary increases, higher positions, academic productivity as measured by publications and scholarship income should be defined and evaluated in mentoring programs, which is unfortunately in most studies not the case. Mentoring without sponsoring has been shown to improve the mentees' satisfaction, but it is unlikely to bring the mentee into a higher position. Female leadership styles and role models are genuinely different from men but more suitable and more successful for modern working environments. Without clear perspectives, without structural changes, female mentees will, despite their knowledge, skills, and networks, continue to lag behind their male colleagues when it comes to promotion and leadership careers. Our society must not miss out on the important opportunities for renewal and sustainability that would come with highly motivated and talented female leaders.

Mentoring programs must therefore have clear definitions of success and must involve all individuals, male and female, at all levels, and especially senior male leaders who still hold most of the positions of power today. To ensure the success of mentoring, structural changes are necessary. The literature supports a binding quota for women in leadership positions to avoid stereotype female assignment and role struggle for these women. Only if women appear as a group and not as the single female in a male group will women in leadership not have to face and struggle with the issue of being a woman but will be seen for their expertise and skill. We should embrace the change in leadership style women bring as important resource and bring them to action. Instead of training women to assimilate to male leadership styles and role models, mentoring programs should encourage women to pursue this different leadership style and to become a different role model, which is more suitable for modern institutions.

Mentoring programs should affirm women to dare to be different from men, to combine improvement in self-confidence and resilience with teaching leadership know-how, for example, difficult conversations, raising visibility, how to negotiate, grant application, and research skills. Future female leaders should be made aware of pink-on-pink aggression and should be instructed and motivated as part of mentoring programs to stop and sanction this detrimental behavior as it is widespread and can have a negative impact on female careers. As part of mentoring, mentees themselves should develop a thorough understanding of diversity and inclusion, considering them future leaders that implement and live diversity and inclusion in their future institution. We must keep in mind that privilege is invisible to the one who holds it. Therefore, to create a true understanding of inequality through direct personal experience, senior male colleagues should be involved as mentors in female mentoring programs.

Mentoring provides tailored advice, whereas a sponsor has power and is willing to use it for his or her mentee. Only if mentoring is combined with sponsoring can real career opportunities for the mentee be created and only then mentoring programs can reach their dedicated goal of bringing more women into leadership. This implies also involving senior male mentors in female mentoring programs as still today they are the ones holding most positions of power. Program design should take this into consideration but also evaluate this concept.

Again, it is useful to look back at history: the goddess Athena—a female figure—had to repeatedly slip into the male guise of mentor to assist her protégé Odysseus and his son and ultimately broker peace with the inhabitants of Ithaca.

In the twenty-first century, we should be more advanced and give power to the numerous competent women. We should be open for new leadership styles and role models introduced by women and reassure them to lead differently. Mentoring programs must be well-designed and include sponsorship to bring women into leadership positions that help ensure success and sustainability of companies and institutions worldwide.

7.14 Summary

Mentoring programs alone do not bring more women into leadership positions. Sponsoring is a must.

Society needs to work on actively placing women in positions with power, accepting that female quotas are an important step to make women seen for their skill not their gender.

To achieve this, male-dominated structures must be broken up, old role models questioned, and leadership styles rethought.

Only with these combined measures can mentoring programs lose their fig-leaf character and have a lasting, successful impact on women's careers.

References

1. Kang SK, Kaplan S. Working toward gender diversity and inclusion in medicine: myths and solutions. Lancet. 2019;393(10171):579–86. https://doi.org/10.1016/S0140-6736(18)33138-6.
2. Burkhart S (2021) Warum Mentorin bei Frauen nicht wirkt. Available from: https://steffiburkhart.com/warum-mentoring-bei-frauen-nicht-wirkt/. Accessed 28 Feb 2025.
3. Statistisches Bundesamt available at: Heft_91_Homepage_Stand_07_10_2024.pdf. Accessed 8 Mar 2025.
4. Homer (ca. 750 v.Chr.): Odyssee.
5. Ziegler A. Mentoring: Konzeptuelle Grundlagen und Wirksamkeitsanalyse. In: Stöger Heidrun (Hrg.), Mentoring: Theoretische Hintergründe, empirische Befunde und praktische Anwendungen. Lengerich: Pabst; 2009. p. 7–30.
6. Sambunjak D, Straus SE, Marusić A. Mentoring in academic medicine: a systematic review. JAMA. 2006;296(9):1103–15. https://doi.org/10.1001/jama.296.9.1103.
7. House A, Dracup N, Burkinshaw P, Ward V, Bryant LD. Mentoring as an intervention to promote gender equality in academic medicine: a systematic review. BMJ Open. 2021;11(1):e040355. https://doi.org/10.1136/bmjopen-2020-040355.
8. Vassallo A, Walker K, Georgousakis M, Joshi R. Do mentoring programmes influence women's careers in the health and medical research sector? A mixed-methods evaluation of Australia's Franklin Women Mentoring Programme. BMJ Open. 2021;11(10):e052560. https://doi.org/10.1136/bmjopen-2021-052560.
9. Laver KE, Prichard IJ, Cations M, Osenk I, Govin K, Coveney JD. A systematic review of interventions to support the careers of women in academic medicine and other disciplines. BMJ Open. 2018;8(3):e020380. https://doi.org/10.1136/bmjopen-2017-020380.
10. Grisso JA, Sammel MD, Rubenstein AH, Speck RM, Conant EF, Scott P, Tuton LW, Westring AF, Friedman S, Abbuhl SB. A randomized controlled trial to improve the success of women assistant professors. J Womens Health (Larchmt). 2017;26(5):571–9. https://doi.org/10.1089/jwh.2016.6025. Epub 2017 Feb 28
11. Kaiser CR, Major B, Jurcevic I, Dover TL, Brady LM, Shapiro JR. Presumed fair: ironic effects of organizational diversity structures. J Pers Soc Psychol. 2013;104(3):504–19. https://doi.org/10.1037/a0030838. Epub 2012 Nov 19
12. Eagly AH, Carli LL. Through the labyrinth: the truth about how women become leaders. Boston: Harvard Business Review Press; 2007.

13. Teresa Victoria. Talk "Pink on Pink Aggression". Boston Children's Hospital, Harvard Medical School 2024.
14. Gokli A, Kaplan SL, Victoria T. Recognizing and mitigating female-to-female aggression in professional settings. Pediatr Radiol. 2024;54(12):2082–5. https://doi.org/10.1007/s00247-024-06062-9. Epub 2024 Oct 2
15. Mitchell P. How to mentor and support other women—and help them succeed. March 6, 2020. Available at: https://ideas.ted.com/how-to-mentor-and-support-other-women-and-help-them-succeed/. Accessed 28 Feb 2025.
16. Harris C. How to find the person who can help you get ahead at work. November 2018. Available at: https://www.ted.com/talks/carla_harris_how_to_find_the_person_who_can_help_you_get_ahead_at_work. Accessed 28 Feb 2020.

Women in Clinical and Academic Medicine, How to Enable Well-Being, and Train Resilience

8

Eva Schönefeld and Bettina Pfleiderer

The WHO constitution states: "Health is a state of complete physical, mental and social well-being and not merely the absence of disease or infirmity." An important implication of this definition is that mental health is more than just the absence of mental disorders or disabilities (https://www.who.int/data/gho/data/major-themes/health-and-well-being).

8.1 Background

Since the 1940s, the concept of stress as a health risk factor was introduced by Selye, a physician (Selye) [1]. Since the 1990s, stress has been increasingly identified as an undesirable condition for medical and academic female professionals in the medical field [2–6]. A lack of well-being of medical and academic professionals due to stress leads to acute and chronic diseases, and even to a reduced life expectancy [3]. This chapter will help better understand and recognize stress and stressors to optimize stress management to improve the well-being of physicians and academic professionals

Stress constitutes an individually perceived burden of physical and mental challenges that depends on individual responses, team or working circumstances, and institutional and societal frameworks. Stress is counterproductive to well-being and

E. Schönefeld (✉)
Institute of Medical Education and Students' Affairs, Medical Faculty University of Muenster, Münster, Germany
e-mail: eschoene@uni-muenster.de

B. Pfleiderer
Research Group Cognition & Gender, Clinic of Radiology, Münster, Germany
e-mail: pfleide@uni-muenster.de

S. Keller-Yamamura, J. Yamamura (eds.), *Inclusive Radiology: Fostering Diversity and Equity in Academic and non-Academic Settings*,
https://doi.org/10.1007/978-3-032-05705-1_8

involves an individual dose- and perception-dependent response pattern that can be modified through training.

In his book *Calm and Confident on Stress* [1], G. Kaluza presented three components of stressors that triggers stress as a health risk factor:

1. The first component includes external stressors such as the given environmental framework or circumstances.
2. The second component relates to individual stress amplifiers.
3. The third component depends on personal and physical reactions on stress.

His work is considered one of the most influential and profound concepts of stress. According to him, some components of individual stress response patterns can be reduced or modified through individual or group training. There are also components of stress that are difficult to change. These are mostly related to structural or organizational frameworks or even socialization.

8.2 Stress and Stressors

Psychosocial stressors have a negative impact on well-being and resilience [4–8]. It is essential to be aware of these factors and how to modify them [9–11]. In 1994, American psychiatrists [4] working on sexual harassment noted that in medicine, especially academic medicine, psychosocial stressors have an impact on three different levels:

First, they identified study- or work-related stressors; for example, time management in surgery [4–7]. In this context, there are also individual personality factors such as perfection. Within their meta-analysis, the perfection factor appeared to be an index factor in medicine that could lead to stress [4, 7, 12, 13].

Second, women in medicine and academia are at a high risk to experience stress. This was explained by social and lower female self-esteem self-worth [4]. Social psychologists have confirmed this observation by analyzing group dynamics in terms of power and agency [14]. Because of stereotypes about women and the associated expectations that they should form attachments and be primarily responsible for maintaining relationships, there is a discrepancy for women to take on more power and agency, even to be more aggressive in a convenient but necessary way. This is not in line with their social role [3, 4, 13, 14]. Stereotypes are generalized judgments that categorize individuals on the basis of incomplete knowledge about the social groups to which others think they belong, leading to certain expectations about their behavior and abilities [12].

Third, another factor that may influence psychosocial stress of women in academic and/or medicine is the institutional framework and policies, which often offer a guiding principle of gender equality, although women's daily experiences contradict this principle.

Psychosocial stressors have a negative impact on well-being and may lead to burnout symptoms [2] in a dose- and perceptual-manner. Women have a higher risk of suffering from psychological stressors [2]. Since the 1990s, a great deal of research has been done to understand stress and health concepts for physicians [3–8]. Most stressors are comparable across all fields in medicine, even though there are some specific factors such as in surgery.

Preventive interventions have recently been introduced into medical education [9, 10]. Students are trained to be able to develop resilience.

The following presents several stressors. The list is not exhaustive.

General stressors [2]:

- Organizational challenges in the workplace
- Lack of optimal information, sources, and communication
- Regulatory overload (complexity and flexibility)
- Hierarchy
- Abuse of power and influence by perpetrators
- Loss of teamwork
- Social issues
- Gender, especially queer identities
- Minorities
- Patients´ health as a priority
- Lack of medical training in self-reflection and self-care
- Value that self-care is a deficit or a weakness

Based on literature [3–5, 15], we would suggest an additional list of psychological stressors that are mainly impacting women negatively:

Female stressors:

- Sexual discrimination and violence [5]
- Sexual harassment [5]
- Discrepancy between the stereotype of a managerial position and being a woman
- Still being a minority, especially in leadership positions
- Lower agency as a stereotype
- Assumed higher risk of female radiologists´ when being pregnant; maternity protection conditions lead to longer periods of training as junior physician
- Reduction to her appearance (style or beauty) rather than competence
- Simultaneous and more caring responsibilities than men
- Patients' attitudes and behavior toward female professionals
- Prejudices, stereotypes, and their reinforcement in the workplace
- Putting hard-earned success at risk

Latest research highlighted that implicit gender bias negatively impacts women's life expectancy in the United States. [4]

8.3 Acute and Chronic Reactions to Stress

> Stress reactions cause a general activation, which shows itself in characteristic changes of physical functions, of thoughts and feelings and in behaviour. [2]

Stress may result in *acute emotional and physical reactions*. Emotions are regulated in the limbic system of the brain, resulting in, for example, anxiety, nervousness, and hasty behavior. Depending on biographical experiences, the reactions may be positively linked on some levels [1].

Blood circulation in the brain is increased, salivation is reduced, and pain tolerance is temporarily increased. The brain is the assessment and control center for all further reactions and reflexes. From the evolutionary perspective, we are activated for fight or flight. Breathing rate increases, bronchial dilatation occurs. Faster heart rate and increased blood pressure can occur. All these signs are observable and be useful for resilience training. Muscle tension increases and reflexes improve. Sweating may occur and energy supply is required through an increased blood sugar and activated fats. On the other hand, the digestive activity is reduced and energy storage is inhibited. Blood clotting is increased. Cold hands and feet can be observed. Libido is inhibited while immune competence is increased in the short-term. In Fig. 8.1, the consequences of acute and chronic stress are illustrated.

If the *stress persists* for a longer period of time, it is known that our brain is shaped, and mental disorders can occur. Emotionally, empathy is reduced, exhaustion occurs, and burnout symptoms may lead to loss of motivation, resignation from

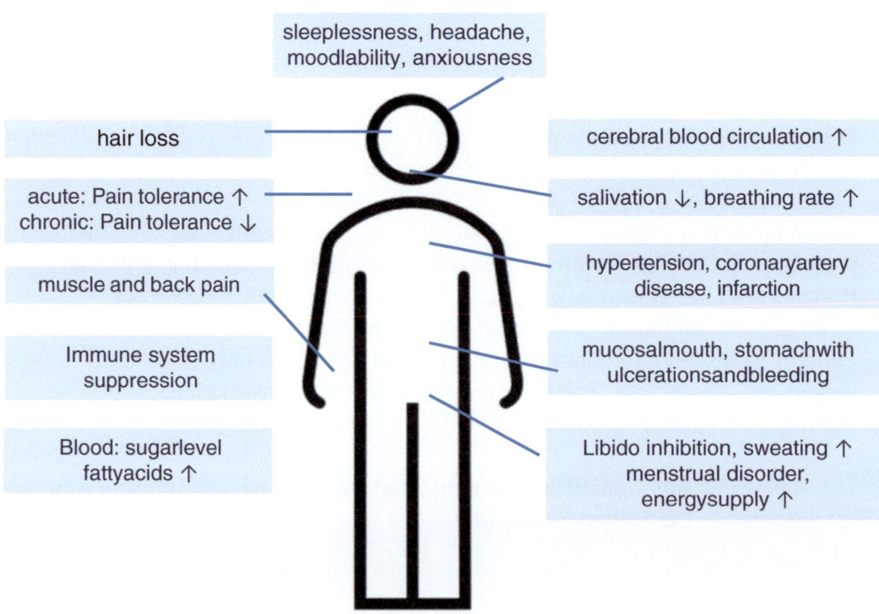

Fig. 8.1 Illustration concerning acute and chronic stress reactions

work or even the medical profession. There are several studies and surveys from the 1990s [3, 4] that have led to preventive ambitions for healthcare workers. *Stress depression* is the umbrella term for mental disorders and impaired cognitive and memory functions. At least, chronic stress leads to cerebrovascular diseases, including cerebral infarction and hypertension-dependent cardiovascular diseases, especially for women [6].

The loss of female physicians within the labor market and the physicians´ own illnesses should give more attention to well-being and prevention through resilience training.

Chronic stress [1]: The hypothalamus–pituitary–adrenal cortex axis remains permanently activated. The stress brake (cortisol release) is switched off and there are permanently higher levels of cortisol in the blood. This has complex effects on the organ systems and diabetes, for example, can occur. In addition to depression, there are various other psychological symptoms such as anxiety. Coping strategies to deal with stress can also be risky, for example, smoking or alcohol consumption.

The brain is also affected by impairment in memory function and cognitive performance. Cerebral infarction may be a long-term consequence. There may be increased intraocular pressure, tinnitus, or sudden deafness. Chronic hypertension can lead to coronary heart disease, atherosclerosis, and heart attack.

Other known symptoms of chronic stress include headache, back pain, various orthopedic entities, and soft tissue disorders. Digestive disorders and gastrointestinal ulcers are reported, as well as an increased prevalence of cancer. The immune system is weakened in the long term, leading to increased health risks. Autoimmune reactions are observed. Pain tolerance is reduced, libido loss, cycle disorders, and even infertility.

8.4 Interventions

It is a general principle of life to be aware of a balanced mixture of tension (stress) and relaxation [1]. Stress reactions are individual and based on biographical experiences. Nevertheless, stress has an impact on physical and mental health [2–8]. In particular, the high quality and complex demands of work in the health and the academic sectors put self-observation or self-reflection at risk. There is a need for training in the appropriate management of stress and modifiable stressors [8]. One should be aware of physical reactions to specific situations that are included in the acute stress reactions above.

Example 8.1

How do you feel and react when a patient dies? How do I feel and what are my physical symptoms when giving a patient a fatal prognosis or illness? What is my time management ability in general? Do I often work overtime?

The first step to deal with stress is to *recognize* it. This is self-monitoring: What are my personal physical reactions or signals due to stress? Being aware of one's symptoms, one is given the ability to act against the negative influence. Even thoughts before the stress incidence occurs may help you to reduce your reaction to it. The goal of observing one's stress reactions, physical symptoms, or one's mental strain offers the possibility of more sensitivity and awareness, on the one hand, and more resilience in the long run.

If this seems to be too difficult, professional support may be indicated: from coaches, counselors, or psychotherapists. Even the Jacobson muscle relaxation technique is an option that can be implemented in one's daily work.

The second step in dealing with stress and its symptoms is, according to the *Berking model for training emotional competency and resilience* [16], visualizing them: After observing one's emotions and symptoms, they should be *named*, written down, for example, in a diary, and communicated about them with close friends. Naming and sharing can provide initial relief and perspective.

A third step may be to search for *self-support*.

Example 8.2
What helps me to recover? How do I recover? Do I take time out for my hobbies, for example, sport, reading books? Are my basic needs met? Am I tired and in need for sleep? Am I hungry?

The fourth step is *social contact*. Talk with some close friends or a supportive person (coach, supervisor, etc.) about your observations and challenges as well as your need of self-support. With repeated practice, you will become more aware of your individual situations and your individual physical reactions and patterns. In addition, social contact has a key role to play through empathy, validation, and empowerment if the right people are chosen for support.

After training and social support, it would be helpful to develop your plan and go into *confrontation with alternative reaction patterns*. Professional counseling may be useful to increase one's competence at this point.

Example 8.3
If you are experiencing physical symptoms such as an increased heart rate and/or breathing rate or neck pain starts, a breathing exercise [10] could be helpful. It can be observed that a well-trained breathing exercise leads to reduced heart rate, emotional downregulation, and several other positive effects.

These steps, according to the model of Berking [16], aim at a higher level of resilience and positive effects on stress management, both individually and/or in professional contact. Stress reduction can be achieved through a variety of exercises and focusing on breathing is known by meditation, and it is necessary to find the individual focus and exercise that is most supportive. Frequent practice increases resilience [11].

Preventive measures are increasingly being implemented already in medical education [9, 10]. Several clinical institutions offer mental and physical health programs and questionnaires [11–13], while recognizing that exhaustion and stress among medical professionals results in loss to the labor market [5–7]. Neuroscience provides insights into healthy coping strategies, although more work is needed [11].

References

1. Kaluza G. Calm and confident on stress. Heidelberg: Springer; 1991. https://link.springer.com/book/10.1007/978-3-662-64440-9.
2. Wittchen HU, Hoyer J. Klinische Psychologie & Psychotherapie, vol. 1131. Heidelberg: Springer; 2011. p. 136–7.
3. Cunningham JB, Wicker P. Sexual harassment and implicit gender career biases negatively impact women's life expectancy in the US: a state-level analysis, 2011–2019. BMC Public Health. 2024;24:1115. https://doi.org/10.1186/s12889-024-18450-9.
4. Charney DA, Russell RC. An overview of sexual harassment. Am J Psychiatry. 1994;151:10–7.
5. Bergner T. Lebensaufgabe statt Lebens-Aufgabe: Burnout bei Ärzten. Dtsch Arztebl. 2004;101(33):A2232–4. (German).
6. Wilkinson E. UK NHS staff: stressed, exhausted, burnt out. Lancet. 2015;385:841.
7. Von dem Knesebeck O, Klein J, Grosse Frie K, et al. Psychosocial stress among hospital doctors in surgical fields. Dtsch Arztebl Int. 2010;107(14):248–53. https://doi.org/10.3238/arztebl.2010.0248.
8. Cohen JS, Patten S. Well-being in residency training: a survey examining resident physician satisfaction both within and outside of residency training and mental health in Alberta. BMC Med Educ. 2005;5:21. https://doi.org/10.1186/1472-6920-5-21.
9. Warnken I, Polujanski S, Rotthoff T, et al. Stress experience and coping strategies in medical studies – insights and a discussion of preventive measures. GMS J Med Educ. 2025;42(1):Doc6.
10. Brinkhaus B, Stöckigt B, Witt CM, et al. Reducing stress, strengthening resilience and self-care in medical students through Mind-Body Medicine (MBM). GMS J Med Educ. 2025;42(1):Doc7.
11. Regehr C, Glancy D, Pitts A, et al. Interventions to reduce the consequences of stress in physicians – a review and meta-analysis. J Nerv Ment Dis. 2024;202:353–9.
12. Petersen L, Dietz J. Die Bedeutung von Stereotypen und Vorurteilen für das Diversity Management (German). In: Becker M, Seidel A (Hrsg.) Diversity – Unternehmens- und Personalpolitik der Vielfalt. Schäffer-Poeschel; 2006. p. 106–122.
13. Keller M, Bamberg E, Kersten M, et al. Validierung des Instruments zur stressbezogenen Arbeitsanalyse für Klinikärztinnen und -ärzte (ISAK). Zeitschr Arbeit Orga Psychol. 2013;75(1):3–21.
14. König O. Macht in Gruppen – Gruppendynamische Prozesse und Interventionen. München: Pfeiffer bei Klett-Cotta; 1995.
15. https://www.who.int/data/gho/data/major-themes/health-and-well-being
16. Berking M, Wupperman P, Reichardt A, et al. Emotion-regulation skills as a treatment target in psychotherapy. Behav Res Ther. 2008;46(11):1230–7. https://doi.org/10.1016/j.brat.2008.08.005.

Training and Working Conditions in Germany: Insights from Training Surveys

9

Carolin Siech

9.1 Introduction

Residency represents an important milestone for physicians. Since residency is one of the first steps of clinician's career path, the training period is therefore a formative period in which the basic directions for the future career are defined. Training and working conditions of physicians have been the subject of extensive research. Training surveys provide valuable insights into the challenges as well as the opportunities faced by residents and young physicians at the local, national, and international levels. This chapter summarizes the findings of various contemporary training studies and explores how these insights can be leveraged to improve medical training and working conditions for the next generation of physicians. Furthermore, special attention is given to gender-related issues, particularly unconscious discrimination against female physicians in residency training.

Outline: What are the findings from studies on working and training conditions of the next generation of physicians in the national and international context? How can these observations be used to improve the status quo? Which factors need special consideration to avoid unconscious discrimination of minorities and female physicians in residency training?

C. Siech (✉)
Department of Urology, University Hospital, Goethe University Frankfurt, Frankfurt am Main, Germany
e-mail: Siech@med.uni-frankfurt.de

S. Keller-Yamamura, J. Yamamura (eds.), *Inclusive Radiology: Fostering Diversity and Equity in Academic and non-Academic Settings*,
https://doi.org/10.1007/978-3-032-05705-1_9

9.2 Inside Germany: Insights from National Surveys

First evaluations of the German Medical Association (Bundesärztekammer [BÄK]) in 2009 and 2011 have already identified key challenges and areas for improvement regarding training and working conditions for physicians in Germany. Moreover, trainers (Weitebildungsbefugte) were also interviewed by BÄK. However, more recent surveys, such as those conducted by Marburger Bund, Hartmannbund, as well as specialty-specific training surveys initiated by various junior groups of specialist societies and summarized as metanalyses by the Bündnis Junge Ärztinnen und Ärzte (BJÄ), continue to show the shortcomings already described in 2009 and 2011. Unfortunately, these observations indicate that many of the challenges already reported more than 15 years ago persist today. In consequence, addressing these structural issues remains vital for improving training and working conditions for residents in Germany.

9.2.1 Residency Evaluation of the German Medical Association

In 2009 and 2011, the BÄK examined the working and training conditions of physicians in Germany in a uniformly structured manner, identifying key challenges and areas for improvement [1, 2]. Although requiring to answer 100 questions covering eight different question categories, response rates among residents were as high as 33% in 2009 (18,856 residents) and 39% in 2011 (20,518 residents) and provide a solid basis for drawing conclusions about residents on national level in Germany [1, 2]. Using a grading scale from 1 (fully applies) to 6 (does not apply at all), the overall assessment of the training situation was rated on average 2.54 in 2009 [1, 2]. The workplace culture received a rating of 2.13, transfer of specialist knowledge of 2.52, decision-making culture of 2.21, leadership culture of 2.45, and learning culture was assessed at 2.39 [1, 2]. These evaluations showed little variation across different regions and medical specialties. However, university hospitals generally provided better training structures, while smaller hospitals often struggled to meet educational requirements. Addressing working conditions, 92% of respondents reported working overtime, 45% stated that this extra work was partially or not at all documented, and 54% indicated that their overtime was only partially or never compensated through time off or payment [1]. In both surveys, a significant proportion of residents expressed dissatisfaction with their residency programs. One of the main issues reported was the lack of structured mentorship, feedback, and supervision. Only a minority had access to structured training curricula or regular evaluations [1, 2]. Female trainees faced more obstacles in career advancement, including implicit biases and limited access to high-quality training opportunities. Moreover, work–life balance was a significant concern, particularly regarding family planning and parental leave options.

As a result of a broad discussion on the continuation of the residency evaluation of the BÄK and in assessment of the pilot surveys carried out in five medical associations at the state level in 2014, the Executive Board of the BÄK has decided to further conduct the training surveys on a decentralized basis under the responsibility of the individual medical associations using a uniform nationwide core questionnaire. Nonetheless, this decision created a significant knowledge gap. Despite national recommendations by the BÄK, training surveys continued at the state level were inconsistently designed and distributed at different times. These differences render national comparisons impossible.

9.2.2 Marburger Bund Barometer 2021

The Marburger Bund's 2021 survey (MB-Barometer 2021) represents one of the largest contemporary national training surveys in Germany [3]. Involving 3238 residents, MB-Barometer 2021 highlighted widespread dissatisfaction among residents in Germany. The majority of residents were female (62%), had a full-time working position (81%), and were hired at a hospital with more than 400 beds (65%) [3]. Staff shortages were cited as the primary barrier to high-quality training (84%), followed by a lack of structure in residency programs [3]. Only 15% of respondents received a structured training plan, and merely 10% received regular feedback from their trainers [3]. Overall, 62% of participants were dissatisfied with their training situation [3]. These dissatisfaction levels emphasize the urgent need for improved training conditions, particularly through structured training and extended staff recruitment.

9.2.3 Hartmannbund's Residency Survey 2024

Similarly, the recently published Hartmannbund's 2024 survey reinforced these concerns [4]. Of 487 residents, around 70% reported being unable to take legally mandated breaks, and 40% faced challenges in documenting overtime. More than 40% rated their employer's staffing situation as inadequate [4]. Moreover, 36% of respondents had considered leaving the profession due to excessive workload, limited free time, and lack of recognition [4]. Despite the tense personnel situation, most employers do not yet seem to see the need to improve working conditions. Around 86% of respondents have no opportunity to work remotely, only 17% are involved in optimization of processes, and only 24% have offers for stress reduction or prevention by their employer [4]. Hartmannbund's 2024 survey also addressed the area of digitalization. Duplicate documentation is faced by 70% respondents in daily clinical practice. For over 90%, constraints with the IT infrastructure are part of everyday working life. These findings underscore the urgent need for systemic changes and more effort regarding digitalization in German hospitals to improve working conditions for residents.

9.2.4 Specialty-Specific Training Surveys

Specialty-specific training surveys serve as essential tools for assessing the quality, structure, and effectiveness of residency programs across different medical and surgical fields in Germany. Moreover, they allow specialty-specific comparisons between different hospitals and regions. Specialty-specific surveys play a crucial role in identifying strengths and weaknesses, allowing evidence-based improvements, and ensuring that residency programs align with the needs of future specialists and the evolving demands of their field of interest. Additionally, these specialty-specific surveys help in standardizing competency-based training curricula, adapting training structures to evolving healthcare demands and promoting inclusive learning environments. Subject-specific priorities and challenges can be identified. For example, training surveys among residents in general medicine focused on outpatient care experiences, financial support for residents, and rural practice exposure [5]. Findings of training surveys contributed to improvements in funding programs for residency in general medicine. Conversely, the joint surgical training survey of the professional association of German surgeons (BDC) and the Young Surgeons' Perspective Forum of the German Society of Surgery (DGCH), specifically assessed surgical residency conditions, focusing on operating room experience, case variety, and workload distribution [6]. Results have led to more structured supervision and protected training time in surgical disciplines. Last but not least, national training surveys among urologic residents, conducted by the German Society of Residents in Urology (GeSRU), showed a large discrepancy between satisfaction with the choice of specialty (79%) and satisfaction with the current job situation (48%) [7]. Only one in four (23%) participants received a structure for its residency [7]. These observations formed the basis for the structuring and standardization process of urological residency in Germany, resulting in the development of the new training curriculum for urology (Weiterbildungscurriculum Urologie [WECU]) of the German Society of Urology (DGU), together with the Professional Association of Urology (BvDU) and GeSRU [8, 9].

9.2.5 Meta-Analyses of Bündnis Junge Ärztinnen und Ärzte (BJÄ)

Original articles, such as those specialty-specific training surveys described above, provide important insights into training and working conditions of young physicians in Germany. Additionally performed meta-analyses in which the original data are aggregated may offer a more advanced level of evidence. Therefore, BJÄ summarized data from previously published training surveys from six different specialties, namely internal medicine (n = 1696), anesthesiology and intensive care medicine ($n = 848$), urology ($n = 384$), gynecology and obstetrics ($n = 391$), ophthalmology ($n = 221$), and radiology ($n = 501$), as secondary analysis [10]. Among 4041 residents, 60% were female, 35% had children, and 84% were working full-time [10]. Of these, only 46% were satisfied with their current job situation [10]. Around 32% were active in science [10]. Focusing on the model of professional gratification crises by Siegrist [11], the mean effort–reward (ER) ratio was 1.8 ± 1.3, demonstrating an imbalance of psychosocial workload among surveyed residents [10]. Specifically, advanced stage of residency and higher age were both associated with lower job satisfaction and a higher ER ratio [10]. These observations are worrying since an imbalance of effort and reward factors at work might have consequences not only for the junior doctors themselves, but also for the patients they care for [12–14]. A healthy work environment with health professionals in good health is therefore crucial and should be in everyone's interest.

9.3 Beyond Borders: Global Perspective on Training Surveys

International training surveys from Europe as well as North America provide important insights into training and working conditions of high-income countries beyond Germany's national borders. In the following, we provide three examples from the Netherlands, the United States, and Canada.

9.3.1 Insights from the Netherlands

Among 1231 Dutch residents across 33 specialties, van Vendeloo et al. reported a burnout rate of 15% [15]. After adjusting for demographic (age, gender, and marital status) and work-related factors (year of training, type of teaching hospital, and type of specialty), perceived quality of the learning environment was inversely associated with the risk of burnout [15].

9.3.2 Insights from the United States

Evaluating the well-being of 1708 residents across general surgery, internal medicine, and pediatrics programs at 14 academic health systems in the United States, Pololi et al. identified work–life integration, relationships, institutional support, respect, values alignment, and ethical distress as the strongest predictors of resident vitality, together accounting for 50% of vitality variance [16]. Conversely, individual demographics accounted for just 3% of variance [16].

9.3.3 Insights from Canada

Conducted in the province of Alberta, Cohen et al. examined perceived stress levels, mental health status, and the availability of well-being resources [17]. Of 415 residents, 34% reported their life as being stressful, mainly related to time pressure and more frequent in females than males (40 vs. 27%) [17]. If given the opportunity, 14% would change their specialty program and 22% would not pursue medicine [17]. Intimidation and harassment was reported by 55% of residents, strongly related to female sex (38 vs. 12%) [17]. Well-being resources included colleagues (67%), program directors (60%), and external psychiatrist/psychologist (49%) [17].

9.4 Improving the Status Quo: Lessons from Training Surveys

Despite the different time periods and thematic focuses of the aforementioned training surveys, some common conclusions can be drawn and three important measures were derived.

9.4.1 Structured Training Curricula

Contemporary training surveys still indicate that only a minority of residents received a curriculum or a training plan at the beginning of their residency. Although relying on novel competence-oriented training regulations, many residents fear that they will not be able to complete the required content of the training regulations defined by the new "Musterweiterbildungsordnung 2018" (MWBO) within the designated time of residency.

Structured training curricula are critical for trainee development since they ensure high-quality and standardized training considering the limited period of residency. Moreover, training curricula emphasize national comparability, allowing residents to receive skill development across different institutions. This uniformity also facilitates an easier transition between job positions, without facing major disruptions in the learning progress. Furthermore, structured curricula provide planning security for both trainees and trainers, enabling them to set clear expectations regarding training content, timelines, and evaluation criteria. A well-organized curriculum also ensures a comprehensive representation of required training content, covering all essential aspects of a specialty and promoting a broader understanding of the specialty. Additionally, structured training fosters better collaboration between hospital-based and office-based physicians, bridging gaps between outpatient and inpatient care and benefiting both healthcare professionals and patients. Implementing standardized curricula, pilot projects such as the joint residency program in general medicine (Weiterbildungsverbund Allgemeinmedizin) [18] or the training curriculum in urology (Weiterbildugscurriculum Urology [WECU]) can serve as models and provide ideas for other specialist areas [8, 19].

9.4.2 Working Time Regulations, Mentorship, and Support Systems

Contemporary as well as historical training studies indicate that German residents frequently work long hours, often exceeding the legal limit of the European Working Time Directive (EWTD), which limits working hours to 48 hours per week. Many residents reported regularly working beyond this limit, often without proper documentation or compensation of overtime. International comparisons reveal similar patterns, particularly in the United States.

Overcoming these challenges, working time regulations have been implemented not only at the legislative level but also through collective bargaining between employers and the physician's trade union in recent years. To enhance work–life balance, it is necessary to better enforce existing working time regulations. In current bargaining agreements, both number of shifts and on-call duties per month as well as working hours on weekends are limited. Additionally, the implementation of effective monitoring systems, such as electronic time tracking system, can help reduce excessive workloads.

Excessive workloads and inadequate compensation contribute to burnout, job dissatisfaction, and a decline in work–life balance. Burnout, mental health concerns, and psychosocial workload are prevalent among residents worldwide. A recurring theme in training surveys is the variability in supervision and the lack of mentorship. Similarly, annual training meetings defined in the training regulations rarely take place. In Germany, as in many other countries, the availability of structured mentorship programs is inconsistent.

Well-structured mentorship correlates with increased job satisfaction, better skill development, and improved mental well-being among residents. Therefore, standardized mentorship programs, including structured feedback mechanisms and at least annual training interviews, should be integrated as a fixed component into residency programs. Best-practice models could serve as a guide. Moreover, a welcoming working atmosphere, social networks, and support programs represent essential components to reduce psychosocial workload and prevent burnout. Supportive social networks may include colleagues, program directors, and external psychiatrist or psychologist.

9.4.3 Equal Opportunities in Career Advancement

Various studies suggest that female physicians face barriers in career progression due to unconscious biases. Training surveys indicate that female trainees are more likely to be assigned administrative or patient communication tasks, while male colleagues receive more procedural training.

Especially in the context of the increasing proportion of women in medicine, equal distribution of training opportunities is essential. Structured evaluation criteria and transparent promotion processes can help mitigate gender disparities. Moreover, medical training structures must adapt to accommodate the diverse needs of residents, including minority groups and physicians with family responsibilities. Family-friendly policies addressing maternity and parental leave as well as flexible working time models are increasingly in demand from both women and men that allow part-time work and parental leave without career disadvantages. Countries such as Sweden have successfully implemented flexible remote working models. Examples include digital consultations in primary healthcare and rehabilitation [20, 21] as well as home visits and virtual medical rounds [22]. Adapting similar models in Germany would enhance inclusivity and should be prioritized to retain as many colleagues as possible in the healthcare system.

9.5 Conclusions

Residents in Germany face significant challenges in medical training and professional practice, particularly due to staff shortages, inadequate training structures, and poor work–life balance. By identifying both strengths and weaknesses in the training process, training surveys can help ensure the quality of residency programs in Germany. Additionally, training surveys provide valuable insights into physician's working conditions, enabling the development of strategies and structural improvements to enhance residency programs.

Amid shortage of medical professionals, training surveys can also help to identify reasons why physicians leave patient care, switch to other professional fields, or migrate abroad. Understanding these factors is crucial for implementing necessary reforms to continuously improve residency programs. Targeted measures include structured training curricula, working time regulations, mentorship, and support systems, as well as equal opportunities in career advancement. These elements form the foundation for comprehensive reforms aimed at retaining medical professionals within the healthcare system while enhancing the overall training and working environment. Ultimately, such comprehensive improvements will make the medical profession more attractive for future generations.

Literature

1. Bundesärztekammer. Ergebnisse der Evaluation der Weiterbildung—1. Befragungsrunde 2009—Bundesrapport 2009.
2. Bundesärztekammer. Ergebnisse der Evaluation der Weiterbildung—2. Befragungsrunde 2011—Bundesrapport 2011.
3. Marburger Bund. MB-Barometer „Ärztliche Weiterbildung". 2021.
4. Hartmannbund. Assistenzärzt:innen-Umfrage 2024. 2024.
5. Karsch-Völk M, Jäkel K, Schneider A, Rupp A, Hörlein E, Steinhäuser J. Evaluation of GP specialty training in Bavaria - an online survey among postgraduate trainees. Z Für Evidenz Fortbild Qual Im Gesundheitswesen. 2016;113:56–65. https://doi.org/10.1016/j.zefq.2016.04.001.
6. Braun B. Gemeinsame Assistentenumfrage des BDC und des Perspektivforums Junge Chirurgie der DGCH 2018/2019. Passion Chir 2020;2019.
7. Arnold H, Fassbach M, Mattigk A, Zehe V, Beck A, Wundrack F, et al. Weiterbildungs- und Arbeitsbedingungen urologischer Ärztinnen und Ärzte in Weiterbildung in Deutschland. Urol. 2021;60:1025–34. https://doi.org/10.1007/s00120-021-01608-3.
8. Michel MS, Himmler M, Necknig U, Kriegmair M, Speck T, Fichtner J, et al. Zertifiziertes Weiterbildungscurriculum für die Facharztweiterbildung in Urologie der Deutschen Gesellschaft für Urologie gemäß der Musterweiterbildungsordnung 2018 (Fassung vom 20.09.2019). Urol. 2020;59:135–40. https://doi.org/10.1007/s00120-020-01367-7.
9. Leyh H, Faßbach M, Siech C. Zertifiziertes Weiterbildungscurriculum der Deutschen Gesellschaft für Urologie e. V. (WECU). Urol. 2025. https://doi.org/10.1007/s00120-025-02568-8.
10. Joachim SC, Bitzinger D, Arnold H, Lermann J, Oechtering TH, Schott S, et al. Die Arbeits- und Weiterbildungssituation junger Ärztinnen und Ärzte in Deutschland—eine zusammen-

fassende Analyse von Befragungsergebnissen aus sechs Fachrichtungen. Gesundheitswesen. 2020;82:227–35. https://doi.org/10.1055/a-0945-9387.

11. Siegrist J, Wege N, Pühlhofer F, Wahrendorf M. A short generic measure of work stress in the era of globalization: effort-reward imbalance. Int Arch Occup Environ Health. 2009;82:1005–13. https://doi.org/10.1007/s00420-008-0384-3.
12. Vu-Eickmann P, Li J, Müller A, Angerer P, Loerbroks A. Associations of psychosocial working conditions with health outcomes, quality of care and intentions to leave the profession: results from a cross-sectional study among physician assistants in Germany. Int Arch Occup Environ Health. 2018;91:643–54. https://doi.org/10.1007/s00420-018-1309-4.
13. Dragano N, Siegrist J, Nyberg ST, Lunau T, Fransson EI, Alfredsson L, et al. Effort–Reward imbalance at work and incident coronary heart disease: a multicohort study of 90,164 individuals. Epidemiology. 2017;28:619.
14. Wege N, Li J, Siegrist J. Are there gender differences in associations of effort-reward imbalance at work with self-reported doctor-diagnosed depression? Prospective evidence from the German Socio-Economic Panel. Int Arch Occup Environ Health. 2018;91:435–43. https://doi.org/10.1007/s00420-018-1293-8.
15. van Vendeloo SN, Prins DJ, Verheyen CCPM, Prins JT, van den Heijkant F, van der Heijden FMMA, et al. The learning environment and resident burnout: a national study. Perspect Med Educ. 2018; https://doi.org/10.1007/S40037-018-0405-1.
16. Pololi LH, Evans AT, Civian JT, Shea S, Brennan RT. Resident vitality in 34 programs at 14 academic health systems: insights for educating physicians and surgeons for the future. J Surg Educ. 2018;75:1441–51. https://doi.org/10.1016/j.jsurg.2018.04.021.
17. Cohen JS, Patten S. Well-being in residency training: a survey examining resident physician satisfaction both within and outside of residency training and mental health in Alberta. BMC Med Educ. 2005;5:21. https://doi.org/10.1186/1472-6920-5-21.
18. Schwill S, Magez J, Joos S, Steinhäuser J, Ledig T, Rubik A, et al. New paths in post-graduate medical training in general practice - 8 years of experience with the pilot project Verbundweiterbildung(plus) Baden-Württemberg. GMS J Med Educ. 2017;34:Doc62. https://doi.org/10.3205/zma001139.
19. Siech C, García CC, Leyh H, Schmid H-P, Engl TA, Karakiewicz PI, et al. Standardized evaluation of satisfaction within urology residents during clinical training: implementation of a new urological residency rotation program at the university hospital Frankfurt. Front Surg. 2022;9:9.
20. Fernemark H, Skagerström J, Seing I, Ericsson C, Nilsen P. Digital consultations in Swedish primary health care: a qualitative study of physicians' job control, demand and support. BMC Fam Pract. 2020;21:241. https://doi.org/10.1186/s12875-020-01321-8.
21. Qvarfordt M, Nilsson E, Nilsson L. Health care professionals' experiences in telerehabilitation: qualitative content analysis. JMIR Hum Factors. 2023;10:e40690. https://doi.org/10.2196/40690.
22. Fernemark H, Skagerström J, Seing I, Hårdstedt M, Schildmeijer K, Nilsen P. Working conditions in primary healthcare during the COVID-19 pandemic: an interview study with physicians in Sweden. BMJ Open. 2022;12:e055035. https://doi.org/10.1136/bmjopen-2021-055035.

Gender Discrimination: Still a Reality in the 2020s? 10

Isabelle Redenius

In her best-selling book *Invisible Women*, the author Caroline Criado Perez comprehensively summarized in a fact-based manner the effects of explicit and implicit gender bias against women in everyday life [54]. Biases that still exist in the 2020s as numerous publications about "The Gender Pay Gap" [1] and gender stereotypes [2] have shown in recent years.

Stereotypes are, from a psychological perspective, useful. They help us structure the world without requiring constant deliberation, saving brain capacity for other tasks. However, in a professional context, these stereotypes unfortunately subconsciously prevent decisions from being made based on merit alone, thus resulting in disadvantage and discrimination.

One reason for the discrimination against women is the concept of homosociality—the phenomenon that people predominantly associate with individuals of the same gender—which results in the direct disadvantage of women in personnel decisions at the top executive level. Due to affinity bias—a cognitive bias where people particularly like those who are similar to themselves—this decision-making process is strongly influenced by sympathy and antipathy, causing pure professional qualifications to take a back seat [3]. The affinity bias often results in the selection of the person with whom the top decision-makers can identify the most: frequently, this is another man who shares many similarities with them.

According to the affinity bias, people tend to prefer hiring individuals who are similar to themselves. This similarity principle not only results in qualified candidates being overlooked but also leads to the cultivation of increasingly homogenous teams—especially at the top decision-making level that is mostly male-dominated. Such homogeneity extending not only to gender but also to social background,

I. Redenius (✉)
Evidia Medical Care Center (MVZ), Braunschweig, Germany
e-mail: isabelle.redenius@evidia.de

S. Keller-Yamamura, J. Yamamura (eds.), *Inclusive Radiology: Fostering Diversity and Equity in Academic and non-Academic Settings*,
https://doi.org/10.1007/978-3-032-05705-1_10

age and nationality, among other aspect of diversity, imposes a major pitfall: it steadily diminishes the capacity for innovation and with regard to healthcare, fails to address the needs of a diverse population. Homogeneous teams, in turn, often display conformity bias, where differing opinions or contrary approaches are not openly addressed in oder to align with the majority view and avoid standing out negatively. While this may initially seem comfortable for all involved, as consensus in joint decision-making is typically reached more quickly than in heterogeneous teams, it carries the risk that discriminatory and toxic behaviors and practices are less critically questioned and can thus become firmly established.

Another form of gender bias is double standards in evaluations. Assertive women are often perceived as bossy, bitchy, or even aggressive, whereas assertive men are seen as confident, charismatic, and strong in leadership. Women are still expected to ensure harmony. The crux is that when women try to conform to this behavior, they increase the risk of being perceived as weak and, consequently, as unsuitable for leadership positions.

Gender stereotypes have a significant impact on both our private lives and our work lives. Our stereotypical conditioning ensures that we perceive and evaluate the same behaviors and abilities differently in men and women. A man who works part-time for family reasons is met with confusion, while it is accepted for a woman. A woman who works full-time despite having children is seen as surprising, whereas for a man, it is considered normal.

Also to the mentioned is the "beauty is beastly" effect, where women benefit from their appearance and feminine attributes in low-status jobs, but face disadvantages when it comes to high-status professions, such as becoming a doctor or scientist [4]. The reason given for this is the "fatal woman" or "evil seductress" motif. This motif reflects a subconscious fear among people of all genders that attractive women might misuse their appearance to manipulate others, typically men [5]. As a result of this phenomenon, women with strong feminine attributes are often denied their competence. It is important that people—colleagues and patients in regard to female healthcare professionals—start to realize that outward appearances do not allow any conclusions about a person's character, abilities, and professional competence.

Explicit and implicit bias affect the hiring process as well as promotions [6–8] and are experienced throughout the working day: either if it is automatically assuming that a woman is not as strong or capable as a man in physical tasks or interrupting and talking over women in group settings more than men [9]. It has also been investigated that a woman's appearance or behavior is seen more critical compared to a man's [10], again a form of double-standard evaluation.

These biases also affect women in the healthcare sector as has been investigated in numerous publications [11]. It also affects the leadership opportunities where women are often passed over for healthcare leadership positions in favor of male candidates [12]. This is one of many reasons why there is a huge gap in between the number of female medical students and the number of female healthcare leaders. Other reasons, for example, are that women still do more housework, there are insufficient childcare options, childcare is predominantly taken on by mothers, and more women also take on the care of family members. This lack of support for balancing work and family responsibilities due to a lack of flexible work policies in healthcare settings are a major contributor to this gender gap [13].

It is statistically proven that in the winter semester 2022/23 in Germany, 64% of medical students were female; at the same time, however, less than half (49%) of working physicians were female. Among working radiologists, the female proportion was only 37%. When looking at the leadership level, the number of female individuals continues to decrease: out of a total of 14 clinical fields, the number of female senior physicians was 37%, female chief physicians were 19%, and female hospital directors were 13% [14]. Where do all the women disappear?

Ongoing discriminations and nonphysical violence up to harassment and physical threats create a hostile work environment [15], which, in the worst case, can lead to women significantly reducing their working hours or switching to another, non-male-dominated area. Some of these discriminations are unintended, for example, when unknowingly holding biases leads to differential treatment in the workplace [16]. In the surgical and interventional specialties, female doctors face stereotypes that question their physical strength and emotional suitability for these high-pressure environments. Women in healthcare settings may be stereotyped as being less competent or capable than their male colleagues, leading to questioning their assertiveness and decisiveness and resulting in unequal opportunities for advancement [17].

This questioning of female competence affects not only superiors and colleagues but also patients. This might lead to patients questioning a diagnosis and treatment plans or even to a patient's refusal to be treated by a female doctor. A more common scenario is that female doctors are frequently mistaken for nurses or other healthcare staff, which can undermine their authority in the eyes of patients and colleagues.

Even more concerning are jokes, derogatory or suggestive comments, and instances of sexual harassment directed at female employees perpetrated not only by patients but also by colleagues. This crucial issue is discussed in a separate chapter.

In the context of family planning and child-rearing, many gender stereotypes and role expectations persist, with significant consequences also for female healthcare professionals. Women are often presumed to want children, regardless of their actual desires or capabilities. If they do have children, they face criticism no matter their choices: continuing to advance their careers can lead to perceptions of being neglectful mothers, while reducing their work hours to focus on family might result in accusations of lacking professional ambition.

Which male doctor has ever been asked questions like: "What does it feel like to have achieved the position of Chief Physician as a man?" or "When you attend a conference, who takes care of the children?" A woman would hardly be praised for also taking care of their common children, whereas a man is applauded for it. "Wow, I think it's really impressive that your husband takes care of the kids while you're at a refresher training!"—you will rarely find a woman who has heard this sentence the other way around.

Presumably the underlying problem is primarily that mothers are generally seen as a potential risk in the workforce.

The often unspoken argument from companies to avoid hiring women of childbearing age is based on the assumption that they do not want to invest in training a woman, only to later be informed that she will soon go on maternity leave and be absent for several months or even years.

Many workplaces operate under the presumption that as soon as women become mothers, their careers will take a backseat. This often leads to the automatic assumption that women returning from parental leave will only be partially capable and less resilient as they will now primarily focus on their role as mothers.

As a result, mothers are frequently perceived as less ambitious and flexible, and are seen as not having the suitability and necessary conditions for relevant projects and positions [18].

This viewpoint not only discriminates against childless women of childbearing age who cannot or do not want to have children but are nonetheless subjected to a blanket suspicion with resulting negative consequences. It also places immense pressure on those who would like to become mothers without having to accept a career setback. They feel the expectation that, as mothers, they would have to work as if they had no children, while also being expected to raise their children as if they had no job [19]. In deciding for or against children, many career-driven women weigh the potential impact on their careers.

In times of skilled labor shortages, which prevail in many industrialized countries, the prejudiced discrimination against women of childbearing age, along with the resulting professional disadvantages, is also harmful to the economy and society.

The comparatively low employment rate of women represents a significant untapped economic potential in many industrialized societies.

At this point it should also be mentioned that societal expectations to be the sole provider for the family also sometimes weigh heavily on fathers, and the conflict between different role expectations affects men as well. Men who deviate from traditional role expectations, such as taking extended parental leave or stepping back from their careers to care for their children, likewise often encounter skepticism and resistance. Nowadays many fathers consider it ideal if both parents are to a similar extent employed and share the housework and childcare equally [20]. But until now the change has mainly been reflected in a shift in values rather than in actions [21].

Due to societal expectations of gender roles, not only mothers but also fathers who wish to do so find it difficult to take on a larger share of child-rearing responsibilities. In a study commissioned by the Anti-Discrimination Agency of the Federal Republic of Germany, nearly one in three fathers reported derogatory or negative reactions to the announcement of their parental leave [22]. Thus, if we want to achieve greater participation of women in the workforce, there must also be a shift in the stereotypical expectations of men. To counter the aforementioned prejudices and role expectations, these gender stereotypes must be questioned on various levels. This starts with parents and caregivers and continues with teachers and trainers. Gender-stereotypical role models can also be actively challenged through books, educational materials, films, etc. Additionally, the importance of recreational facilities such as sports clubs and coaches should not be underestimated. Companies also play a key role in successfully combating gender-based prejudices. Employees who make personnel decisions within the company should be trained to raise awareness of biases. Leaders should be aware of their responsibilities and use fair and transparent criteria for hiring, promotion, and performance evaluation. Feedback from the workforce, such as through anonymous surveys, is also useful for gaining insights into problematic areas.

Additionally, companies could establish networks for women to facilitate experience exchange and mentoring. For example, the German Radiological Society created the network radiologinnen@drg [23], which serves as a mentoring program among other functions.

Companies should be aware that a lack of diversity in the workforce increases the risk of losing innovation potential and profitability. A McKinsey study from 2020 shows that companies with high gender diversity are 25% more profitable [24]. While profitability should not be the main focus in healthcare, innovation is nonetheless essential. Lastly, political measures such as family policy reforms and initiatives for stereotype-free career and study orientation are needed to dismantle gender stereotypes.

We hinder progress in the equality and diversity debate when we simultaneously expect tolerance and openness while generalizing people based on attributes they cannot control, such as age, skin color, and gender —for instance, in phrases like "old white men. People are not a homogeneous mass. Yes, the debate about equal opportunities is urgently needed, as is the discussion on how to sustainably change the status quo. However, it must not lead to black-and-white thinking by broadly condemning all older white men. Only through cooperative and nuanced dialogue can we successfully advance toward genuine equality, which is essential for a country's future and competitiveness. Together, not against each other.

It cannot be emphasized enough that not only female doctors but also female and transgender patients are victims of discriminations that affects the quality of care that they receive, leaving them misunderstood, mistreated, and misdiagnosed.

It starts with how doctors are trained. Historically, it has been assumed that there was not anything fundamentally different between male and female bodies other than size and reproductive functions, and so for years medical education has been focused on a male "norm" with everything that falls outside that designated "atypical" or even "abnormal" [25].

When women *are* mentioned, they are presented as if they are a variation on standard humanity. Students learn about anatomy and *female* anatomy. Physiology and *female* physiology. *Male* is hardly ever emphasized separately because it is already taken as the norm. Illustrations in textbooks and on posters about "The Muscular System," "The Nervous System," and "The Vascular System" generally feature a large-scale man.

We might shrug at illustrations, but when it comes to the treatment of diseases, the matter becomes serious. Until now there is only minimal integration of sex- and gender-based medicine in med schools, with gaps particularly seen in the therapy of diseases and drug use [26].

We continue to rely on data from studies done on men as if they apply to women. For many calculations, a "standard man" weighing 70 kg (154 pounds) and being 170 cm tall (5′7″) was and is used as a reference to represent humanity as a whole, although it does not even represent men particularly well. Interestingly, the concept of the "Reference Man" was developed by the International Commission on Radiological Protection in 1974 to assist in the estimation and standardization of radiation exposure to individuals [27].

Although meant to represent humanity as a whole, the levels of radiation that are safe for "Reference Man" turn out to be anything but for women. Women exposed to ionizing radiation during childhood suffer from cancer at a rate 10 times higher than predicted by traditional models used by the United States Nuclear Regulatory Commission. The Use of Reference Man masks gendered impacts and therefore systematically underreports radiation harm [28].

This is also reflected in clinical studies where historically women have been underrepresented in medical research studies in part due to concerns to involve women in reproductive ages due to the risks for pregnant women and the fetus. Results from clinical trials were presented as valid for men and women even when women were excluded from the study [29]. Interestingly, the proportion of female authorship positively correlates with a higher proportion of women included in clinical trial [30]. However, just as women are underrepresented in clinical studies, they are also significantly underrepresented among the authors of clinical studies [31].

Even today, arguments can be found suggesting that the female body is too variable and complex and thus too costly to be tested on [32]. Females might even not be included in animal studies on female-prevalent diseases [33]. The same applies to cell studies, where even for diseases that occur more frequently in women, there are still more studies using only XY cells [34]. Women are not just smaller men; in fact, female and male bodies differ even on a cellular level, with varying concentrations of many metabolites differing wildly in female and male human cells [35].

As a result, many medical treatments and protocols are based on research done primarily on men, leading to a lack of understanding of how certain conditions or medications affect women differently [36] not taking into account that different immune systems and different hormones can play a role in how chemicals are absorbed or accumulate in women's higher percentage of body fat. Researchers have found sex-based differences in every tissue and organ system in the human body [37], as well as in the prevalence, progression, and severity of the majority of common human diseases [38].

This lack of female representation in clinical research studies leads to a lack of gender-specific treatment options for women [39]. It raises the question how many treatments women might have missed out on because they had no effect on the male cells on which they were exclusively tested.

On the other hand, this can result in treatments and medications that are less effective or have more side effects for women [40] and can even have life-threatening consequences: the antidepressant fluvoxamine results in up to 100% higher blood levels in women at the same dose compared to men, significantly increasing the risk of overdose. Similarly, with certain sedatives, the U.S. Food and Drug Administration had to subsequently reduce the dosage for women by half after it was found that the medication demonstrably shortened women's lives [41].

Despite clear sex differences, the vast majority of drugs, including anesthetics and chemotherapeutics, are still administered with gender-neutral dosages, putting women at risk of overdose or underdose [42]. This one-size-fits-all approach, based on male-dominated clinical trials, is likely to be a major cause for women being more likely to suffer adverse drug reactions than men [43]. Researchers have found a drug dose gender gap for 86 different medications approved by the Federal Drug Administration (FDA), including antidepressants, cardiovascular, and anti-seizure drugs and analgesics, among others [44]. Even most generic drugs have "statistically significant differences between men and women in bioequivalence" compared with reference drugs [45].

Regarding the treatment of pregnant women, we lack solid data for almost anything, although the WHO warns that many diseases can have "particularly serious consequences for pregnant women, or can harm the foetus." [46] When it comes to treatment options, sex differences affect not just medical therapy. In a 2014 review about a cardiac resynchronization therapy device, it was found that the threshold to have a CRT-D implanted was set too high for women [47], raising the question how many heart failures could have been prevented in female patients.

Gender discrimination is not only about the data gap due to the lack of research, including both sexes and transgender people. It is also about the social meaning that was and still is ascribed to the female body. There is a known gender bias in pain management where female patients' pain is taken less seriously than that of male patients or how coronary heart disease is diagnosed and treated [48]. A female patient might be prescribed a less effective or lower dosage of medication compared to a male patient with the same condition due to the assumption that women may not tolerate certain treatments as well as men [49].

Biases in communication or decision-making inadvertently disadvantage women in their healthcare experiences. Women are dismissed or not taken seriously by healthcare providers when reporting symptoms or seeking medical help, leading to delayed or misdiagnosed conditions, such as heart disease or autoimmune disorders [50], as well as pain assessment and mental health disorders [51]. Making assumptions about a woman's health based on stereotypes or prejudices results even nowadays in paying less attention to women's complaints and dismissing women's concerns or symptoms as being exaggerated or psychosomatic compared to men's. As a consequence, this may lead to delayed or inadequate treatment and providing lower quality care to women [52]. The gender bias might even go as far as assuming that a woman is not the primary decision-maker in her own healthcare choices and deferring to a male family member instead [53].

The lack of correct diagnosis and treatment for certain medical conditions has its origin in an androcentric worldview that considers the focus on men as the social norm. In this worldview, maleness (as well as whiteness) is implicit and does not need to be vocalized; because male is the norm, it is presumed to be objective and even universal. This male universality is also a cause of the gender data gap: because male data makes up the majority of what we know, what is male comes to be seen as universal. It leads to the positioning of women, half the global populations, as a minority and as a deviation from standard humanity [54].

When it comes to diseases that primarily affect women, such as pelvic-floor health, breast cancer, or reproductive health, there is a lack of funding compared to research on male-centric diseases [55]. One of the causes can be the lack of representation in healthcare leadership: women are underrepresented in positions of power within the healthcare industry, which can lead to policies and decisions that do not adequately address women's health needs. Overall, addressing these forms of discrimination requires a concerted effort to ensure gender-equitable treatment and representation in healthcare settings, both in research and clinical practice. The question, "Why is gender a factor?", is waiting for researchers to tackle [56].

Especially in regard to the emerging use of AI systems in the medical world to guide diagnoses, we have to make sure to close the medical data gap when it comes to women. Otherwise, AI could make diagnosis for women worse, rather than better.

It is the twenty-first century. The medical world needs to wake up. Both in terms of the gender data gap in medical research and with regard to equality and diversity in the workplace.

References

1. American Association of University Women. The simple truth about the gender pay gap.
2. Grandey AA, Furst-Holloway LM. Gender stereotypes in the workplace: the case of emotional labor.
3. Annahita E. von Quotenfrauen und alten weißen Männer Schluss mit Vorurteilen in der Arbeitswelt; 2023, S. 159.
4. Heinman ME, Saruwatari LR. When beauty is beastly: die effects of appearamce and sex on evoluation of job applicants for managerial and nonmanagerial jobs. Org Behav Human Perform. 1979;23:360–72.
5. https://ww.spiegel.de/karriere/diversity-frauen-schönheit-im-job-a-d9d21dbb-8441-4fdb-bd06-88488a706ee3.
6. Sapienza P, Giuliano P. Gender discrimination in hiring: evidence from 19 countries. 2015.
7. Gender bias in the workplace: Why assuming a woman is less qualified is harmful and unjust. Harvard Business Review.
8. Breaking through the glass ceiling: How stereotypes about female competence hold women back in the workplace. J Appl Psychol.
9. https://www.cmu.edu/news/stories/archives/2020/october/women-interrupted-debate.html
10. Rhode DL. The beauty bias: the injustice of appearance in life and law.
11. Winkel AF, Telzak B, Shaw J, et al. The role of gender in careers in medicine: a systematic review and thematic synthesis of qualitative literature. J Gen Intern Med. 2021;36:2392–9. https://doi.org/10.1007/s11606-021-06836-z.
12. Pincha Baduge MSDS, et al. Barriers to advancing women nurses in healthcare leadership: a systematic review and meta-synthesis. eClinicalMedicine. 2024;67:102354. https://doi.org/10.1016/j.eclinm.2023.102354.
13. ALobaid AM, Gosling CM, Khasawneh E, McKenna L, Williams B. Challenges faced by female healthcare professionals in the workforce: a scoping review. J Multidiscip Healthc.

2020;13:681–91. https://doi.org/10.2147/JMDH.S254922. PMID: 32821112; PMCID: PMC74179.
14. www.statistica.com. Statistic of the Bundesärztekammer.
15. Nelson S, et al. A gender-based review of workplace violence amongst the global health workforce—A scoping review of the literature. 2024. https://doi.org/10.1371/journal.pgph.0003336.
16. Gerull KM, Loe M, Seiler K, McAllister J, Salles A. Assessing gender bias in qualitative evaluations of surgical residents. Am J Surg. 2019;217:306–13.
17. Teede HJ. Advancing women in medical leadership. Med J Aust. 2019;211(e1):392–4. https://doi.org/10.5694/mja2.50287.
18. Kleiner C, Lott Y. Arbeitszeitoptionen im Lebensverlauf, p_wsi_studies_4_2016.pdf (boeckler.de), S. 75.
19. Esmailzadeh A. von Quotenfrauen und alten weißen Männer Schluss mit Vorurteilen in der Arbeitswelt; 2023, S. 159.
20. Institut für Demoskopie Allensbach. Veränderungen der gesellschaftlichen Rahmenbedingungen für die Familienpolitik. 2019.
21. https://www.zeit.de/gesellschaft/familie/2023-02/vaterschaft-alltag-arbeitsteilung-familie-gleichberechtigung-studie
22. https://www.antidiskriminierungsstelle.de/SharedDocs/aktuelles/DE/2022/20220524_Caregiverstudie.html
23. https://www.diversity.drg.de/de-DE/10349/radiologinnen-drg/
24. https://www.mckinsey.de/news/presse/2020-05-19-diversity-wins
25. Marts SA, Keitt S. Principles of Sex-based Differences in Physiology: Foreword: a historical overview of advocacy for research in sex based biology. Adv Mol Cell Biol. 2004;34:1–333.
26. Song MM, Jones BG, Casanova RA. Auditing sex-and gender-based medicine (SGBM) content I medical school curriculum: a student scholar model. Biol Sex Differ. 2016;7(Suppl 1):40.
27. ICRP. Report of the task group on reference man. ICRP Publication 23. Oxford: Pergamon Press; 1975.
28. http://www.passblue.com/2017/07/05/females-exposed-to-nuclear-radiation-are-far-likelier-than-males-to-suffer-harm/
29. Dijkstra AF, Verdonk P, Lagro-Janssen ALM. Gender bias in medical textbooks: examples from coronary heart disease, depression, alcohol abuse and pharmacology. Med Educ. 2008;42(10):2021–8.
30. Chhaya VY, et al. Gender bias in clinical trial enrollment: female authorship matters. Ann Vasc Surg. 2023;95:233–43.
31. Lohana AC, et al. A systematic review of gender disparity in the authorship of clinical trials and clinical practice guidelines in various medicine subspecialties. Cureus. 2024;16(2):e54165. https://doi.org/10.7759/cureus.54165. PMID: 38496166; PMCID: PMC10.
32. Ibarra M, Vázquez M, Fagiolino P. Sex effect on average bioequivalence. Clin Ther. 2017;39(1):23–33.
33. https://thinkprogress.org/scientists-avoid-studying-womens-bodies-because-they-get-periods-3fe9d6c39268/
34. Ortona E, Delunardo F, Baggio G, Malorni W. A sex and gender perspective in medicine: a new mandatory challenge for human health. Ann Ist Super Sanità. 2016;52(2):146–8.
35. Pollitzer E. Cell sex matters. Nature. 2013;500:23–4.
36. Mauvais-Jarvis F. Sex differences in metabolic homeostasis, diabetes, and obesity. Biol Sex Differ. 2015;6:14.
37. Keitt SK, Fagan TF, Marts SA. Understanding sex differences in environmental health: a thought leaders' roundtable. Environ Health Perspect. 2004;112(5):604–9.
38. National Academies Press (US). Why Diverse Representation in Clinical Research Matters and the Current State of Representation within the Clinical Research Ecosystem. 2022 May 17. https://www.ncbi.nlm.nih.gov/books/NBK584396/.
39. Gender bias in clinical trials: implications for women's health. J Clin Pharmacol. 2017;57(6).

40. Carey JL, et al. Drugs and medical devices: adverse events and the impact on women's health. Clin Ther. 2017;39(1):10–22. https://doi.org/10.1016/j.clinthera.2016.12.009. Epub 2017 Jan 7. PMID: 28069260; PMCID: PMC5779632.
41. Weinberger AH, et al. Inclusion of women and gender-specific analyses in randomized clinical trials of treatments for depression.
42. https://www.hindawi.com/journals/bmri/2011/187103/
43. Lack of females in drug dose trials leads to overmedicated women. ScienceDaily.
44. Zucker I, Prendergast BJ. Sex differences in pharmacokinetics predict adverse drug reactions in women. Biol Sex Differ. 2020;11:32. https://doi.org/10.1186/s13293-020-00308-5.
45. Mergaert L, Lombardo E. Resistance to implementing gender mainstreaming in EU research policy. In: Weiner E, MacRae H, editors. The persistent invisibility of gender in EU policy. European Integration online Papers; 2014.
46. http://www.wpro.who.int/topics/gender:issues/Takingsexandgernderintoaccount.pdf
47. Zusterzeel R, et al. Cardiac resynchronization therapy in women: US Food and Drug Administration meta-analysis of patient-level data. JAMA Intern Med. 2014;174(8):1340–8.
48. Beery TA. Gender bias in the diagnosis and treatment of coronary artery disease. Heart Lung. 1995;24(6):427–35. https://doi.org/10.1016/s0147-9563(95)80020-4.
49. Gender disparities in cardiovascular medication use: the role of healthcare providers' biases. J Women's Health. 2020.
50. https://www.escardio.org/The-ESC/Advocacy/women-and-cardiovascular-disease
51. Samulowitz A, et al. "Brave men" and "emotional women": a theory-guided literature review on gender bias in health care and gendered norms towards patients with chronic pain. Pain Res Manag. 2018;2018:1.
52. Zhang L, et al. Gender biases in estimation of others' pain. J Pain. 2021;22(9):1048–59. https://doi.org/10.1016/j.jpain.2021.03.001. Epub 2021 Mar 5. PMID: 33684539; PMCID: PMC8827218.
53. Idris IB, Hamis AA, Bukhori ABM, et al. Women's autonomy in healthcare decision making: a systematic review. BMC Womens Health. 2023;23:643. https://doi.org/10.1186/s12905-023-02792-4.
54. Caroline Criado Perez. Invisible women. 2019.
55. https://www.nature.com/immersive/d41586-023-01475-2/index.html
56. Tackling biases in clinical trials to ensure diverse representation and effective outcomes. Nat Commun. 2024;15:1407. https://doi.org/10.1038/s41467-024-45718-w.

Sexual Harassment in Medicine

11

Bettina Pfleiderer and Eva Schönefeld

Sexual harassment in the workplace occurs every day all over the world: it is a global issue that is still prevalent and a taboo [1]

11.1 Background

11.1.1 Definitions

Workplace violence such as sexual harassment is a hidden pandemic at the workplace globally, and talking about it is still a taboo [1], with women at high risk of experiencing sexual harassment, leading to a reduction in life expectancy [2]. While definitions of sexual harassment may vary, all definitions emphasize the humiliating nature based on an individual's sex. For example, the United Nations defines sexual harassment as *"Sexual harassment is any unwelcome conduct of a sexual nature that might reasonably be expected or be perceived to cause offense or humiliation, when such conduct interferes with work, is made a condition of employment or creates an intimidating, hostile or offensive work environment. Sexual harassment may occur in the workplace or in connection with work. While typically involving a pattern of conduct, sexual harassment may take the form of a single incident"* [3].

B. Pfleiderer (✉)
Research Group Cognition & Gender, Clinic of Radiology, Münster, Germany
e-mail: pfleide@uni-muenster.de

E. Schönefeld
Institute of Medical Education and Students' Affairs, Medical Faculty University of Münster, Münster, Germany
e-mail: eschoene@uni-muenster.de

S. Keller-Yamamura, J. Yamamura (eds.), *Inclusive Radiology: Fostering Diversity and Equity in Academic and non-Academic Settings*,
https://doi.org/10.1007/978-3-032-05705-1_11

In this chapter, we use the definition of the World Health Organization (WHO) [4] because it has a broader scope. Sexual misconduct is an umbrella term according to the WHO definition that contains sexual exploitation, sexual abuse, sexual harassment, and all forms of prohibited sexual behavior. *Sexual harassment* is defined as follows*:*

> *Sexual harassment* is any unwelcome conduct of a sexual nature that might reasonably be expected or be perceived to cause offense or humiliation, when such conduct interferes with work, is made a condition of employment, or creates an intimidating, hostile, or offensive work or operational environment. Sexual harassment may involve any conduct of a verbal, nonverbal, or physical nature, including written and electronic communications, and may occur between persons of the same or different genders [4].

11.2 Forms of Sexual Harassment

Forms of sexual harassment are manifold; in this chapter, we will present the most common forms as presented by the WHO [4] and other research (e.g., 5) (Fig. 11.1).

According to the UN, specific other examples of sexual harassment may also include [3]*:*

- Attempted or actual sexual assault, including rape.
- Sharing or displaying sexually inappropriate images or videos in any format.
- Sending sexually suggestive communications in any format.
- Making inappropriate sexual gestures, such as pelvic thrusts.
- Unwelcome touching, including pinching, patting, rubbing, or purposefully brushing up.

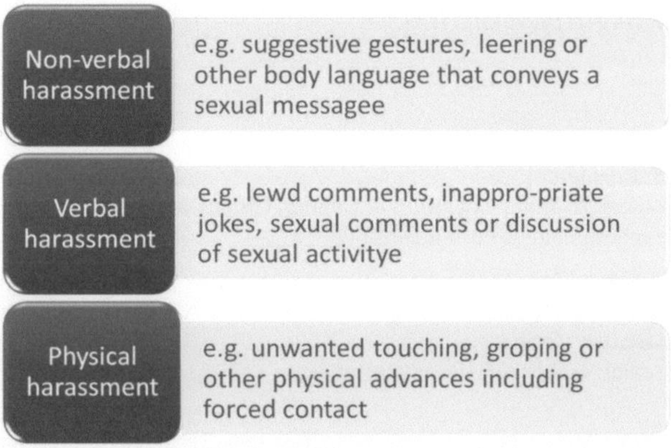

Fig. 11.1 Forms of sexual harassment [4, 5]

- Staring in a sexually suggestive manner.
- Repeatedly asking a person for dates or asking for sex.
- Rating a person's sexuality.
- Making sexual comments about appearance, clothing, or body parts.
- Name-calling or using slurs with a gender/sexual connotation.
- Making derogatory or demeaning comments about someone's sexual orientation or gender identity.

Atypical Sexual Harassment
Another less common but still significant form of sexual harassment is *atypical sexual harassment*. Atypical sexual harassment is sexual harassment where women are sexually harassed by women and men are sexually harassed by women or men [6]. When men are sexually harassed by women, the main types of harassment are verbal and less frequently physical [7]. Very few men report incidents of sexual harassment because they are concerned about being seen as "strong man" if they refuse sexual advances [8].

11.3 Legal Aspects Related to Sexual Harassment

The legal aspects of sexual harassment involve a complex framework of laws, regulations, and policies designed to prevent, address, and remedy instances of harassment in the workplace, including in health and medical settings. These legal standards are critical to holding individuals and institutions accountable for preventing and addressing sexual harassment. They involve definitions regarding sexual harassment, key legislation and legal protections, reporting (internal, external reporting) and related implications, employer and institutional responsibilities (e.g., preventive measures), prevention and training requirements. For these legal frameworks to be effective, they must be supported by comprehensive policies, training, and a culture of zero tolerance for harassment.

Specific legal definitions may vary from country to country. Here, we present three different exemplary frameworks by which sexual harassment can be sanctioned in Germany:

1. Definitions from the *German Penal Code*

"The Penal Code in Germany starts with an antidiscrimination statement: Prohibition of Discrimination Under *Civil Law*: Any discrimination on the grounds of race or ethnic origin, sex, religion, disability, age, or sexual orientation shall be illegal when founding, executing, or terminating civil-law obligations, and further refers to employer.

Penal Law: Enforcement:[1]

(a) Where a breach of the prohibition of discrimination occurs, the disadvantaged person may, regardless of further claims being asserted, demand that the discriminatory conduct be stopped. Where other discrimination is to be feared, he or she may sue for an injunction.
(b) Where a violation of the prohibition of discrimination occurs, the person responsible for committing the discrimination shall be obligated to compensate for any damage arising therefrom. This shall not apply where the person committing the discrimination is not responsible for the breach of duty. The person suffering discrimination may demand appropriate compensation in money for the damage, however not for economic loss.
(c) Claims in tort shall remain unaffected.
(d) The person responsible for committing the discrimination shall not be permitted to refer to an agreement which derogates from the prohibition of discrimination.
(e) Any claims arising from subsections (a) and (b) must be asserted within a period of 2 months. After the expiry of the time limit, the claim may only be asserted when the disadvantaged person was prevented from meeting the deadline through no fault of their own."

2. *General Act on Equal Treatment* for employees´ safety and anti-discrimination framework in Germany.[2]

Subdivision 2 deals with discrimination and paragraph 3 and 4 refers to harassment and sexual harassment as the following citation shows:

> (3) Harassment is deemed to be discrimination when unwanted conduct in connection with any of the grounds referred to in section 1 takes place with the purpose or effect of violating the dignity of the person concerned and of creating an intimidating, hostile, degrading, humiliating or offensive environment.
>
> (4) Sexual harassment is deemed to be discrimination in relation to section 2 (1) nos. 1 to 4, when unwanted conduct of a sexual nature, including unwanted sexual acts and requests to carry out sexual acts, physical contact of a sexual nature, comments of a sexual nature, as well as the unwanted showing or public exhibition of pornographic images, takes place with the purpose or effect of violating the dignity of the person concerned, in particular where it creates an intimidating, hostile, degrading, humiliating or offensive environment.

[1] Sections 177 and 184 of the German Criminal Code (StGB) deal with sexual violence and sexual harassment: https://www.gesetze-im-internet.de/englisch_stgb/englisch_stgb.html

[2] https://www.gesetze-im-internet.de/englisch_agg/englisch_agg.pdf

3. University Frameworks and Codes of Conduct

Students are protected by the local framework at each German university; for example, at the University of Münster:[3]

- Treating each other with respect and appreciation.
- Recognizing and addressing misconduct as well as learning from mistakes.
- Understanding diversity and equality as an asset and opportunity.

11.4 Sexual Harassment in the Workplace

Generally, young people, women, and university staff are particularly affected by sexual harassment in the workplace, resulting often in a "toxic" working environment. The causes of sexual harassment in the workplace seem to be related to unequal power relations [9], social gender roles (Chap. 13), biases and stereotypes (see Sect. 11.4.3), and tolerance of society of certain types of behavior. The problem is exacerbated by a lack of information about support services and inadequate legal consequences [8].

11.4.1 Sexual Harassment in the Medical Sector

Not amazingly, medical trainees experience a high rate of sexual harassment [10]. Already in the 1990s, it was published by Charney and Russell [11] that sexual harassment is also a pervasive problem in the medical and academic sector, which has often been overlooked. Reasons for sexual harassment in the medical workplace include the close working relationship between residents and attending physicians, long shifts, and high-stress working places such as the emergency room, operating rooms, and intensive care units [10]. A German study reported that 76% of female and 62% of male junior physicians experienced sexual harassment when working at the hospital, mostly from colleagues, supervisors, or patients [12]. Another study also shared female physicians being at a high risk to be harassed by patients [13]. These results are in line with a meta-analysis from 2014, showing that 59.4% of medical trainees experienced at least one form of harassment or discrimination during their training with verbal harassment was the most common form [14]. Supervisors were most often the perpetrators, followed by patients or patients' families (34.4% and 21.9%, respectively). A similar report was shared from Finland [15].

Sexual Harassment in Radiology

Sexual harassment has been observed in radiology as well [16–18]. In a survey in 2016, 40% of women and 1% of men reported having experienced sexual harassment in the workplace in a national survey of radiology [16] ranging from inappropriate comments to more serious forms of misconduct. Approximately 10% of

[3] https://www.uni-muenster.de/imperia/md/content/wwu/compliance/code_of_conduct_university_of_muenster_en.pdf

radiologists and radiology trainees are reported to experience sexual harassment, with women more frequently experiencing it [16, 18]. Moreover, female radiologists are more likely to be witnesses of sexual harassment. However, they are less likely to report it [18].

It has been argued that in addition to high-stress situations and hierarchical power structures, radiology faces as an additional risk factor the limited face-to-face interaction, which may increase the challenges of sexual harassment identification, management, and prevention. As in other medical specialties, the number of women in radiology decreases when moving up the career ladder [19], which may be another factor contributing to the challenges tackling sexual harassment in the field of radiology. However, available literature on this topic is scarce and most papers have been based on American data [17, 18].

11.4.2 Sexual Harassment in Medical Education

> Unwanted physical contact and forced physical contact, were perpetrated mainly by patients, whereas sexual assault was perpetrated mainly by superiors and trainers. This suggests that different educational strategies may be needed, targeting patients, staff and supervisors, rather than just fellow students [5].

While women are still underrepresented in medical leadership positions, the number of female trainees and female medical students is increasing, which contributes to the existing gendered power imbalance [5, 9]. Not surprisingly, most victims of sexual harassment, for example, in German medical undergraduates, are female, with [5, 9] verbal and physical sexual harassment experienced the most often [5]. Patients were involved in 19.3% of cases, trainers/supervisors (9.8%), or colleagues (9.3%) in almost 10% of cases [5]. This was corroborated by other studies [20–22]. It was reported that medical graduate students (clinical part) had the highest risk to experience sexual harassment [20].

11.4.3 The Role of Unconscious Gendered Biases and Stereotypes

Biases and stereotypes play a significant role in both the presence and persistence of sexual harassment in the workplace and more so in medicine (Chap. 13). These social perceptions about others often shape the way individuals are treated, the way behaviors are interpreted, and how power dynamics play out in the workplace.

> *Implicit gender bias* is the automatic, unintentional associations that people make about others, such as women in the workplace, and the judgments they make about them, such as good or bad. Implicit biases are automatically activated [2, 23].

Stereotype: Generalized judgments categorizing individuals based on incomplete knowledge about social groups others believe they belong to, leading to certain expectations about their behavior and abilities [24].

It has been shown that sexual harassment combined with unconscious gendered career biases, for example, bias against women working, can reduce the life expectancy of women [2]. Implicit (unconscious) biases can occur due to information overload, low informative value, need for quick decisions, and diversity of information. In a hierarchical workplace such as medicine and academia, biases can create an environment in which sexual harassment is normalized, overlooked, or even tacitly condoned. Implicit biases may lead to a preference for male candidates or senior medical professionals.

The relationship between bias/stereotypes and sexual harassment is complex; a few of the biases/stereotypes that may play a role are.

1. *Stereotypes:*
   - *Picture of a tough hero-like physician*: A pervasive stereotype posits that physicians, particularly male ones, should embody characteristics such as authority, control, and dominance. This stereotype can create an environment where individuals in positions of authority feel entitled to disregard boundaries and engage in inappropriate behaviors without fear of repercussions.
   - *Female subordination*: In certain medical settings, women may be expected to conform to traditional feminine roles, such as nurturing and subservience. This dynamic can render them susceptible to objectification or harassment by male colleagues, who may perceive their submissive behavior as a vulnerability to be exploited for their own benefit, thereby creating an unhealthy power imbalance.
2. *Bias in Reporting and Response to Harassment*
   Biases also affect how sexual harassment is reported, acknowledged, and responded to in the medical field. This can influence whether complaints are taken seriously or dismissed.
   - *Victim blaming* is characterized by the attribution of the victim's responsibility for what had happened. This tendency manifests particularly in instances where the harasser occupies a position of power. For instance, a female medical student or resident might be viewed as "overreacting" or as overly sensitive, based on stereotypes that women are more emotional or less resilient. This dynamic can lead to a reluctance among individuals to report harassment, resulting in an environment where victims may feel isolated or unsupported.
   - *Stereotypical roles of men and women*: The perpetuation of stereotypical roles between men and women contributes to a societal environment that fosters harassment. Furthermore, biases can also manifest in how harassment is perceived based on the gender of the harasser and the victim. In male-dominated medical environments, male colleagues' behavior might be dis-

missed as "joking" or "harmless," while similar actions by women may be viewed more critically.

3. *Cultural and Institutional Norms*
   Hierarchical structures in medicine can make it difficult for those at lower levels (such as students or junior residents) to report harassment or challenge authority figs [9].

11.5 Impact of Sexual Harassment on Health and Well-being

Sexual harassment can reduce a person's competencies to superficial criteria (e.g., dressing) or unchangeable criteria of a person, such as skin color, eyes, sexual orientation, together with negative connotations or devaluing [5]. Not surprisingly, verbal or nonverbal harassment is often associated with emotional abuse and social isolation.

It has also been highlighted that sexual harassment has a negative psychological, professional, and emotional impact on victims [1, 2, 5, 15, 25, 26] and is a *major stressor* negatively impacting health and individual well-being. The effects of stress on health and the human body, as well as the measures to mitigate them, are discussed in detail in Chap. 8.

The health effects may include:

1. *Mental health effects*: anxiety, depression, post-traumatic stress disorder (PTSD [27]) in cases of physical sexual harassment, low self-esteem and self-doubt, feeling of shame and guilt [2, 22, 25, 26].
2. *Physical health effects*: sleep disturbances, somatic symptoms (e.g., headaches), gastrointestinal distress (e.g., nausea, stomach pains), muscle tension, or chronic pain; see increased risk of substance abuse ([22, 25],Chap. 8).
3. *Impact on professional well-being*: burnout, decreased job satisfaction and productivity, withdrawing from colleagues and isolation [22].
4. *Impact on work relationships and social support*: erosion of trust and fear of retaliation, strained interactions with colleagues, supervisors, and even patients [22, 26].
5. *Long-term psychological and physical health effects*: chronic depression [26] and anxiety, reduced life expectancy [2].
6. *Institutional and societal consequences*: for example, high turnover in the healthcare sector, cause individuals to leave their profession or specialty, contributing to workforce shortages [8, 14, 22].

11.6 Addressing and Preventing Sexual Harassment in Medicine

Addressing and preventing sexual harassment in medicine requires a multifaceted approach that includes changes at the individual, institutional, and cultural levels. Given the hierarchical structure of the medical environment and the often-power imbalance between different roles, it is crucial to create a culture of accountability, education, and support, promoting cultural change within academic institutions to prevent future abuse [12]. Below are the strategies and recommendations to help address and prevent sexual harassment in medicine [4, 8, 9, 28].

1. Clear Policies and Reporting Mechanisms [4]
   Clear, accessible, and enforced policies are essential in dealing with sexual harassment. These policies should outline what constitutes sexual harassment, the consequences for perpetrators, and the steps to be taken if harassment occurs. Key components include:
   - *Zero-tolerance policy*: Medical institutions must adopt a clear zero-tolerance policy on sexual harassment, ensuring that any form of harassment is unequivocally condemned and that perpetrators face appropriate consequences.
   - *Confidential and accessible reporting mechanisms*: Institutions should provide accessible, anonymous, and confidential channels for individuals to report harassment without fear of retaliation. This may include hotlines, online reporting systems, or a designated office or officer responsible for handling complaints.
   - *Protection from retaliation*: Victims and witnesses of harassment must be assured that they will be protected from retaliation. Retaliation can take many forms, including career setbacks, social isolation, or informal punishment, and should be strictly prohibited and actively monitored.
   - *Clear and transparent investigation procedures*: There must be a defined process for investigating complaints of sexual harassment that is impartial, confidential, and expeditious. Institutions should ensure that allegations are investigated promptly and fairly, while maintaining transparency to build confidence in the system.
2. Training
   Training is vital for raising awareness and preventing harassment in medical environments. Medical institutions should implement mandatory comprehensive training programs for staff and students:
   - *Mandatory training for all employees and medical students* [9]**:**
     - This training should address:
       - What constitutes sexual harassment.
       - How to recognize subtle forms of harassment (e.g., microaggressions, inappropriate comments).
       - The importance of respecting boundaries and professional behavior.

    - How to report incidents and support affected colleagues.
    - How to intervene if you observe sexual harassment.
    - Culture and bias training.
3. *Ongoing Monitoring and Evaluation* [9]
   Preventing and addressing sexual harassment requires continuous effort and ongoing evaluation. Institutions should establish mechanisms to monitor and evaluate the effectiveness of their anti-harassment initiatives:
   - *Regular surveys and feedback*: Institutions should conduct regular surveys and solicit feedback from staff, students, and trainees to assess the prevalence of sexual harassment, the effectiveness of training programs, and the adequacy of reporting mechanisms. This feedback can be used to refine strategies and policies.
   - *Continuous improvement*: Based on survey results and feedback, institutions should continuously improve policies, training, and support systems. Regular updating and revision of policies ensures that the institution remains responsive to emerging challenges and trends in harassment prevention.

11.7 Conclusion

Sexual harassment is an often-overlooked problem in the medical and academic sectors. Sexual harassment can create a toxic environment that can negatively affect both victims and patients. Medical institutions must ensure a safe and respectful workplace for all individuals by setting policies, training, and monitoring the implementation of measures to facilitate a cultural change.

References

1. Chirico F, Heponiemi T, Pavlova M, Zaffina S, Magnavita N. Psychosocial risk prevention in a global occupational health perspective. A descriptive analysis. Int J Environ Res Public Health. 2019;16(14):2470. https://doi.org/10.3390/ijerph16142470.
2. Cunningham GB, Wicker P. Sexual harassment and implicit gender-career biases negatively impact women's life expectancy in the US: a state-level analysis, 2011–2019. BMC Public Health. 2024;24(1):1115. https://doi.org/10.1186/s12889-024-18450-9.
3. UN System Model Policy on Sexual Harassment. 2023. Retrieved from: https://unsceb.org/sites/default/files/imported_files/UN%20System%20Model%20Policy%20on%20Sexual%20Harassment_FINAL_0.pdf. Accessed 20 Feb 2025.
4. WHO Policy on Preventing and Addressing Sexual Misconduct (PASM). WHO. 2023. Retrieved from: https://cdn.who.int/media/docs/default-source/campaigns-and-initiatives/prseah/who-policy-on-preventing-and-addressing-sexual-misconduct.pdf?sfvrsn=7bb1dd5b_28. Accessed 20 Feb 2025.
5. Schoenefeld E, Marschall B, Paul B, Ahrens H, Sensmeier J, Coles J, et al. Medical education too: sexual harassment within the educational context of medicine—insights of undergraduates. BMC Med Educ. 2021;21(1):81. https://doi.org/10.1186/s12909-021-02497-y.

6. Torres A, Costa D, Sant'Ana H, Coelho B, Sousa I. Sexual harassment and bullying in the workplace in Portugal. Policy Brief. 2016; https://doi.org/10.13140/RG.2.2.32237.69608.
7. McDonald P, Charlesworth S. Workplace sexual harassment at the margins. Work Employ Soc. 2016;30(1):118–34. https://doi.org/10.1177/0950017014564615.
8. Hoel H, Varta M. Bullying and sexual harassment at the workplace, in public spaces, and in political life in the EU. 2018. Contract No.: European Institute for Gender Equality. Lithuania. Retrieved from https://coilink.org/20.500.12592/28p364 on 30 Mar 2025. COI: 20.500.12592/28p364. Accessed 20 Feb 2025.
9. Ludwig S, Jenner S, Berger R, Tappert S, Kurmeyer C, Oertelt-Prigione S, et al. Perceptions of lecturers and students regarding discriminatory experiences and sexual harassment in academic medicine—results from a faculty-wide quantitative study. BMC Med Educ. 2024;24(1):447. https://doi.org/10.1186/s12909-024-05094-x.
10. Komaromy M, Bindman AB, Haber RJ, Sande MA. Sexual harassment in medical training. NEJM. 1993;328(5):322–6. https://doi.org/10.1056/NEJM199302043280507.
11. Charney DA, Russell RC. An overview of sexual harassment. Am J Psychiatry. 1994;151(1):10–7. https://doi.org/10.1176/ajp.151.1.10.
12. Jenner S, Djermester P, Prügl J, Kurmeyer C, Oertelt-Prigione S. Prevalence of sexual harassment in academic medicine. JAMA Int Med. 2019;179(1):108–11. https://doi.org/10.1001/jama.2020.1810.
13. Phillips SP, Schneider MS. Sexual harassment of female doctors by patients. NEJM. 1993;329(26):1936–9. https://doi.org/10.1056/NEJM199312233292607.
14. Fnais N, Soobiah C, Chen MH, Lillie E, Perrier L, Tashkhandi M, et al. Harassment and discrimination in medical training: a systematic review and meta-analysis. Acad Med. 2014;89(5):817–27. https://doi.org/10.1097/acm.0000000000000200.
15. Rautio A, Sunnari V, Nuutinen M, Laitala M. Mistreatment of university students most common during medical studies. BMC Med Educ. 2005;5:1–12. https://doi.org/10.1186/1472-6920-5-36.
16. Perumalswami CR, Jagsi R. Sexual harassment in radiology: prevalence and opportunities for improvement. JACR. 2020;17(2):298–303. https://doi.org/10.1016/j.jacr.2019.09.012.
17. Pitot MA, White MA, Edney E, Mogensen MA, Solberg A, Kattapuram T, et al. You too? Female radiologists' narratives on discrimination and harassment. JACR. 2022;19(2, Part A):288–303. https://doi.org/10.1016/j.jacr.2021.09.043.
18. Camargo A, Liu L, Yousem DM. Sexual harassment in radiology. JACR. 2017;14(8):1094–9. https://doi.org/10.1016/j.jacr.2017.02.054.
19. Cayón Somacarrera S, Alonso Rodríguez C, del Campo Del Val L, Oleaga Zufiría L, Rodríguez Carnero P. Women in radiology: a perspective from Spain. Radiología (English Edition). 2024;66(2):121–31. https://doi.org/10.1016/j.rxeng.2023.04.009.
20. Mahurin HM, Garrett J, Notaro E, Pascoe V, Stevenson PA, DeNiro KL, et al. Sexual harassment from patient to medical student: a cross-sectional survey. BMC Med Educ. 2022;22(1):824. https://doi.org/10.1186/s12909-022-03914-6.
21. Mathews B, Bismark MM. Sexual harassment in the medical profession: legal and ethical responsibilities. MJA. 2015;203(4):189–92. https://doi.org/10.5694/mja15.00336.
22. Menon A. Sexism and sexual harassment in medicine: unraveling the web. J Gen Intern Med. 2020;35(4):1302–3. https://doi.org/10.1007/s11606-019-05589-0.
23. Vuletich HA, Payne BK. Stability and change in implicit bias. Psychol Sci. 2019;30(6):854–62. https://doi.org/10.1177/0956797619844270.
24. Ulloa JG, Viramontes O, Ryan G, Wells K, Maggard-Gibbons M, Moreno G. Perceptual and structural facilitators and barriers to becoming a surgeon: a qualitative study of African American and Latino surgeons. Acad Med. 2018;93(9):1326–34. https://doi.org/10.1097/ACM.0000000000002282.

25. Richman JA, Rospenda KM, Nawyn SJ, Flaherty JA, Fendrich M, Drum ML, et al. Sexual harassment and generalized workplace abuse among university employees: prevalence and mental health correlates. Am J Public Health. 1999;89(3):358–63.
26. Houle JN, Staff J, Mortimer JT, Uggen C, Blackstone A. The impact of sexual harassment on depressive symptoms during the early occupational career. Soc Men Health. 2011;1(2):89–105. https://doi.org/10.1177/2156869311416827.
27. Fitzgerald LF, Hulin CL, Drasgow F. The antecedents and consequences of sexual harassment in organizations: an integrated model. In: Keita GP, Hurrell Jr JJ, editors. Job stress in a changing workforce: investigating gender, diversity, and family issues. American Psychological Association; 1994. p. 55–73. https://doi.org/10.1037/10165-004.
28. Jenner SC, Djermester P, Oertelt-Prigione S. Prevention strategies for sexual harassment in academic medicine: a qualitative study. J Interpers Violence. 2022;37(5-6):NP2490–515. https://doi.org/10.1177/0886260520903130.

Part III

Patient Care and Clinical Work in Health Care and Radiology

Gender Differences in Diagnostic Radiology Practice: Impact on Work Quality and Team Diversity

12

Sarah Keller-Yamamura

12.1 Introduction

While essential to modern medicine, diagnostic radiology reflects gender-specific trends in professional practice that have implications for quality of care, team dynamics, and organizational diversity. By examining the differences in performance, self-assessment, and patient outcomes between male and female radiologists, this chapter explores how such variations underscore the necessity of gender-diverse teams for optimal results.

12.2 Gender-Based Differences in Diagnostic Radiology Practices

Studies reveal that men and women often approach radiological practice differently, influenced by psychological, educational, and cultural factors. Research by Alcaide-Leon et al. highlighted key distinctions in the scope of practice, frequency of seeking second opinions, and error rates among male and female radiologists [1].

Female radiologists tend to exhibit a narrower scope of practice than their male counterparts, often focusing on fewer subspecialties. According to a retrospective study on European teleradiology providers, only 14% of female radiologists reported cases in all three major subspecialties—neurology, musculoskeletal, and body imaging—compared to 27% of male radiologists. Factors such as part-time

S. Keller-Yamamura (✉)
Department of Radiology, Charité-Universitätsmedizin Berlin, Corporate Member of Freie Universität Berlin and Humboldt-Universität zu Berlin, Berlin, Germany
e-mail: sarah.keller@charite.de

S. Keller-Yamamura, J. Yamamura (eds.), *Inclusive Radiology: Fostering Diversity and Equity in Academic and non-Academic Settings*,
https://doi.org/10.1007/978-3-032-05705-1_12

employment, shorter tenure, and preferences for subspecialty work were identified as contributors [1].

Despite a narrower scope, female radiologists demonstrated superior accuracy. The study found that women had a lower adjusted incidence rate ratio (IRR) of errors (0.8) than men, highlighting a meticulous approach to diagnostic imaging. Additionally, while female radiologists were more likely to request second opinions, this tendency was interpreted as a collaborative strategy to enhance diagnostic confidence and accuracy [1] (Fig. 12.1).

The gender differences extend beyond diagnostic radiology into interventional practices. A study by Reder et al. published in *European Radiology* in 2023 [2] investigated gender differences in self-assessed performance, stress levels, and catheter handling during training on basic interventional radiology (IR) maneuvers. The experiment involved 64 participants (26 women and 38 men) who were naïve to endovascular procedures. The study explored how gender influences task performance, stress perception, and self-assessment accuracy during IR training. One of the study's key findings was the significant difference in task performance between male and female participants. Female participants took longer to complete all four tasks than their male counterparts, especially in the most challenging task. In this task, which involved navigating the catheter through the right internal carotid artery, women required significantly more time (688 ± 363 seconds vs. 501 ± 230 seconds, $p = 0.02$). In addition, women were more likely to ask for help earlier and more frequently than men. The study revealed that women requested assistance significantly sooner (203 ± 94 seconds vs. 305 ± 142 seconds, $p = 0.049$), particularly

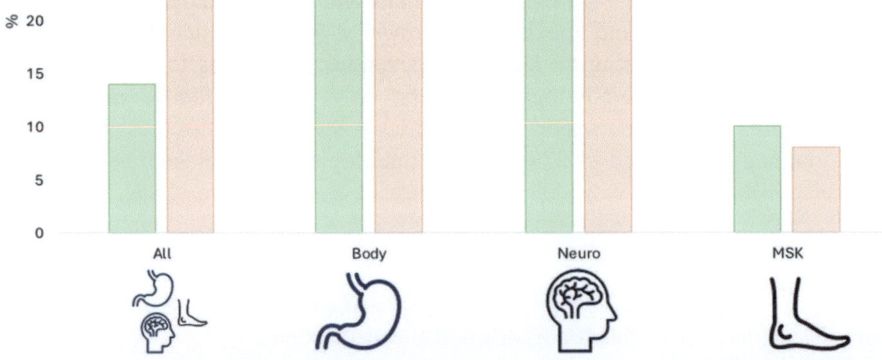

Fig. 12.1 Women have a narrower scope of practice with less overlap (men 27% versus women 14%) in reporting subspecialties. Radiologists were considered to report a subspeciality if more than 1% of their cases belonged to that subspeciality. (Adapted from Alcaide-Leon et al. [1])

during the most complex tasks. Despite these differences, the women in the study were more accurate in self-assessing their performance. They correctly correlated their self-assessment with the objective parameters of the tasks, while the male participants frequently overestimated their performance.

Stress levels were another area where gender differences were observed. Female participants reported higher stress levels (8.9 ± 4.9 vs. 6.3 ± 4.4, $p = 0.037$) and perceived the tasks as more complex (11.5 ± 4.2 vs. 9.6 ± 3.3, $p = 0.016$). This higher level of perceived difficulty and stress could be linked to the observed differences in their approach to task completion. In contrast, the male participants did not show a similar correlation between stress and performance, suggesting that their stress levels may not have influenced their task handling similarly.

Regarding the actual task performance, men displayed more agitated catheter handling, with more movements per second (6.0 ± 1.8 vs. 4.8 ± 1.6, $p = 0.005$). This suggests that men approached the tasks more quickly but with less precision, while women took more time to handle the catheter carefully, possibly to avoid mistakes. As participants were informed about the time tracking of each intervention, it suggests that male participants felt the need to rush because they viewed the experiment as challenging. In contrast, female participants were less competitive and took their time to perform the tasks accurately. This would align with previous reports from Barr et al. on female physicians treating patients with more time, resulting in greater accuracy and patient satisfaction [3, 4]. Women's slower and more methodical approach could contribute to more accurate and controlled task performance despite the longer time required. This strategy may align with research in other medical contexts that shows women tend to perform tasks with more excellent care, potentially reducing complications and enhancing outcomes.

These gender differences in performance, self-assessment, and stress perception have significant implications for training in interventional radiology. The study suggests that gender-specific factors could influence how trainees approach learning tasks and assess their abilities. Female trainees may benefit from support systems that encourage them to trust their skills and reduce stress, while male trainees may need to develop better self-awareness regarding their performance. Additionally, the differences in task handling speed and precision between men and women highlight the importance of tailoring training approaches to accommodate these varying strategies.

Further studies support these findings and found that female physicians are less likely to commit clinically significant errors than men. A comprehensive analysis of Medicare patients revealed that those treated by female physicians had lower 30-day mortality and readmission rates compared to male physicians [5]. Female physicians demonstrated a notable impact on patient outcomes. They achieved a 0.43% reduction in adjusted 30-day mortality rates compared to their male counterparts. Additionally, female-led care resulted in a 0.55% reduction in adjusted 30-day readmission rates. These differences persisted across various conditions and levels of illness severity. The findings align with studies confirming that female physicians adhere more closely to reporting guidelines, contributing to increased accuracy [6, 7] and providing preventive care more often [8, 9]. Above, they tend to spend more time reviewing patient histories and communicating diagnostic results [10], which enhances patient understanding and adherence to treatment plans. This holistic approach reduces immediate readmission rates and fosters long-term health benefits.

Despite all evidence, opinions favoring male physicians based on the assumption that career due to maternity leave, part-time employment, and the additional burden of home responsibilities [11] compromise the quality of care provided by female physicians still exist and are used as arguments toward higher salary for male physicians [12–14].

Gender differences extend far beyond different clinical and interventional medicine performances, influencing factors such as stress and workload perception. Female radiologists in Germany often report higher levels of stress due to additional family responsibilities, with nearly 33% of female participants stating they were primarily responsible for childcare compared to 14% of their male counterparts [15]. It was noted earlier that female radiologists were likelier to report that pursuing academic qualifications, such as an associate professorship, would not be compatible with their family life [15]. While this was not statistically significant, it suggests that the perceived stress of balancing family responsibilities and career ambitions is a concern, especially for women. This highlights how stress perception is intertwined with the demands of academia and family life and may influence women's career decisions. Such disparities underscore the need for organizational policies supporting work–life balance, including flexible schedules and enhanced childcare options.

Interestingly, personality traits also influence stress perception and management. Traits such as conscientiousness and emotional stability correlate positively with reduced burnout and better handling of workload pressures, while neuroticism tends to exacerbate stress responses.

Translating this example of character and personality traits to the interventional study of Reder et al., male participants often underestimated the difficulty of tasks and overestimated their performance. Their stress levels positively correlated with increased agitation and decreased efficiency during challenging tasks. This discrepancy highlights the need for tailored training programs in interventional radiology that address these distinct stress and workload perceptions to optimize learning outcomes [2].

12.3 Gender-Specific Differences in Radiological Research

In research, disparities between male and female radiologists are similarly pronounced. Women often face underrepresentation in authorship positions, particularly in lead roles such as first or last author, which impacts their visibility and career advancement [16–18]. Collaborative networks also play a significant role; men often have more extensive professional networks that facilitate partnerships and increase research output. Conversely, women may encounter challenges in accessing these networks, which limits opportunities for co-authorship and funding acquisition. Balancing work and family responsibilities further compounds these challenges for female radiologists, as time constraints may reduce their ability to engage in intensive research projects. In a recent study [15] on the career development of female radiologists, women ($n = 55$, 33%) stated more frequently than men ($n = 37$, 25%) that pursuing an associate professorship would not be compatible with their family life. However, there was no gender-specific difference in research interest (OR 2.36 (95% CI 1.0–5.57), and interest in teaching (OR 1.86 (95% CI 0.84–4.14)) as a motivator for an associate professorship, implying that external attributors in deed seem to withhold women radiologists from research advancement.

Institutional support, including access to mentorship, funding opportunities, and protected research time, also varies significantly, creating additional hurdles for women. Indeed, women report more often that their gender impacts their institutional support, for example, regarding conference attendance [15]. Despite these challenges, women radiologists have demonstrated significant potential when supported by targeted programs. Mentorship initiatives, especially those fostering diverse mentor–mentee relationships, have been shown to increase research productivity among women. Moreover, institutions adopting flexible working policies and addressing systemic biases have fostered an inclusive environment where female researchers thrive [1].

12.4 Advantages and Challenges of Gender-Diverse Teams

The unique strengths brought by male and female radiologists highlight the importance of diversity in radiological teams. Gender diversity fosters a balanced approach to patient care, problem-solving, and organizational performance. With their meticulous and collaborative tendencies, female radiologists complement the broader scope and higher throughput often associated with male radiologists. This synergy improves patient outcomes, reduces errors, and enhances satisfaction. Furthermore, gender diversity creates inclusive and innovative team dynamics, promoting mutual respect and fostering a collaborative environment.

Nevertheless, challenges persist. Addressing gender imbalances requires targeted efforts to recruit and retain female radiologists, particularly in male-dominated subspecialties such as interventional radiology. Supporting work–life balance through policies like parental leave and flexible work schedules can mitigate career interruptions for women, ensuring equitable advancement opportunities. Mentorship programs address misconceptions and inspire more women to pursue radiology, especially in challenging fields.

The observed differences in radiological practice between men and women reinforce the value of diversity in healthcare teams. By capitalizing on complementary strengths and addressing systemic challenges, the field of diagnostic radiology can achieve superior work quality and patient outcomes. Integrating diverse perspectives at all decision-making levels will improve clinical performance and set a benchmark for equity and excellence in medical practice.

References

1. Alcaide-Leon P, Rawal S, Krings T, Wang G, Zhu J, van Tuijl R, Anderman I, Schorlemmer C. Gender differences in diagnostic radiology practice: an observational study. J Am Coll Radiol. 2022;19(1 Pt A):90–6. https://doi.org/10.1016/j.jacr.2021.09.034. Epub 2021 Nov 9.
2. Reder SR, Rohou A, Keric N, et al. Gender differences in self-assessed performance and stress level during training of basic interventional radiology maneuvers. Eur Radiol. 2024;34:308–17. https://doi.org/10.1007/s00330-023-09993-3.
3. Barr DA. Gender differences in medicine-from medical school to Medicare. Mayo Clin Proc. 2017;92:855–7.
4. Barr DA, Vergun P, Barley SR. Problems in using patient satisfaction data to assess the quality of care provided by primary care physicians. J Clin Outcomes Manag. 2000;7:19–28.
5. Tsugawa Y, Jena AB, Figueroa JF, Orav EJ, Blumenthal DM, Jha AK. Comparison of hospital mortality and readmission rates for Medicare patients treated by male vs female physicians. JAMA Intern Med. 2017;177(2):206–13. https://doi.org/10.1001/jamainternmed.2016.7875.
6. Baumhäkel M, Müller U, Böhm M. Influence of gender of physicians and patients on guideline- recommended treatment of chronic heart failure in a cross-sectional study. Eur J Heart Fail. 2009;11(3):299–30.
7. Roter DL, Hall JA. Physician gender and patient-centered communication: a critical review of empirical research. Annu Rev Public Health. 2004;25:497–519.
8. Andersen MR, Urban N. Physician gender and screening: do patient differences account for differences in mammography use? Women Health. 1997;26(1):29–39.
9. Frank E, Dresner Y, Shani M, Vinker S. The association between physicians' and patients' preventive health practices. CMAJ. 2013;185(8):649–53.
10. Roter DL, Hall JA, Aoki Y. Physician gender effects in medical communication: a meta-analytic review. JAMA. 2002;288(6):756–76.
11. Jolly S, Griffith KA, DeCastro R, Stewart A, Ubel P, Jagsi R. Gender differences in time spent on parenting and domestic responsibilities by high-achieving young physician-researchers. Ann Intern Med. 2014;160(5):344–53.
12. Seabury SA, Chandra A, Jena AB. Trends in the earnings of male and female health care professionals in the United States, 1987 to 2010. JAMA Intern Med. 2013;173(18):1748–50.
13. Nonnemaker L. Women physicians in academic medicine: new insights from cohort studies. N Engl J Med. 2000;342(6):399–405.
14. Jagsi R, Griffith KA, Stewart A, Sambuco D, DeCastro R, Ubel PA. Gender differences in the salaries of physician researchers. JAMA. 2012;307(22):2410–7.
15. Molwitz I, Kemper C, Stahlmann K, Yamamura J, Adam G, Langenbach MC, Reim M, Wegner F, Bannas P, Lotz J, Can E, Zagrosek-Regitz V, Hamm B, Keller-Yamamura S. Gender- and personality-specific differences in academic qualifications, research motivation, and attractiveness of leadership positions: a survey among radiologists from Germany. Rofo. 2024 Oct 16. English, German. https://doi.org/10.1055/a-2415-7337.
16. Piper CL, Scheel JR, Lee CI, Forman HP. Gender trends in radiology authorship: a 35-year analysis. AJR Am J Roentgenol. 2016;206:3–7.
17. Yamamura J, Molwitz I, Ozga AK, Nguyen TA, Wedekind I, Wolf-Baldauf L, Kamo M, Zhao J, Can E, Keller S. Gender differences and cooperation in medical authorships - an analysis of the recent ten years in five key medical disciplines. BMC Med Educ. 2023;23(1):68. https://doi.org/10.1186/s12909-023-04041-6.
18. Molwitz I, Yamamura J, Ozga AK, Wedekind I, Nguyen TA, Wolf L, Kamo M, Zhao J, Can E, Keller S. Gender trends in authorships and publication impact in Academic Radiology-a 10-year perspective. Eur Radiol. 2021;31(12):8887–96. https://doi.org/10.1007/s00330-021-07928-4. Epub 2021 May 19.

The Impact of Unconscious Bias in Healthcare and Diagnostic Imaging 13

Isolde Martina Busch, Michela Rimondini, and Chiara Giraudo

13.1 What Is the Unconscious Bias? Define It to Recognize It

Explicit and implicit biases affect our behavior in different domains, contributing to disparities [1]. For explicit biases, individuals are aware of their prejudices and wrong attitudes toward certain groups being overtly racist, sexist, and homophobic [1, 2].

On the contrary, implicit biases act subconsciously and involve feelings, perceptions, and stereotypes deriving from imprints, previous experiences, and internalized associations between some qualities and specific categories/characteristics, including gender, race, and age [3]. Therefore, individuals act based on prejudice and cliché without being aware or intending it. In 1995, Greenwald and Banaji defined the research domain of "implicit social cognition" and proposed that "*the signature of implicit cognition is that traces of past experience affect some performance, even though the influential earlier experience is not remembered in the usual sense—that is, it is unavailable to self-report or introspection,*" which then produced the concept of implicit bias [4, 5]. Storm and colleagues' review of unconscious bias in human resource management shows that there is still a lack of clear definitions for this concept and no straightforward distinction between the terms "unconscious" and "implicit." Therefore, in the literature, both terms are often used interchangeably [6].

I. M. Busch · M. Rimondini
Department of Neurosciences, Biomedicine, and Movement Sciences, Section of Clinical Psychology, University of Verona, Verona, Italy
e-mail: isoldemartina.busch@univr.it; michela.rimondini@univr.it

C. Giraudo (✉)
Department of Cardiac, Thoracic, Vascular Sciences and Public Health—DCTV, Unit of Advanced Clinical and Translational Imaging, University of Padova, Padova, Italy
e-mail: chiara.giraudo@unipd.it

S. Keller-Yamamura, J. Yamamura (eds.), *Inclusive Radiology: Fostering Diversity and Equity in Academic and non-Academic Settings*,
https://doi.org/10.1007/978-3-032-05705-1_13

Unconscious biases may act at different levels, such as the individual, group, and system/society [6]. At the individual level, some cognitive models define implicit biases as a natural human tendency, and others consider them as elements leading to errors in human judgment and behavior [6, 7]. Within groups, the impact of unconscious biases depends on the categorization of the subjects involved and/or under study, and overall implicit biases guarantee coherence within the group and clear demarcation with those outside [6]. The most frequently investigated unconscious biases at the group level are the gender and the racial ones [6].

Last, at the system/society level, it is a sort of institutionalized bias embedded in such large structures [6].

It is undoubtedly essential to address historical, social, and political factors that influence and shape individual experience [8]. Indeed, it is believed that our biases originate in childhood and are influenced by the reinforcement of social norms, our personal experiences, and those of people in our environment [9]. For instance, regarding race, it has been demonstrated that counties and states in the USA more dependent on slavery in 1860 have more significant implicit pro-white biases among white residents [10]. Regarding gender implicit biases, as highlighted by the 2023 Gender Social Norms Index (GSNI), "*close to 9 out of 10 men and women hold fundamental biases against women. Nearly half the world's people believe that men make better political leaders than women do, and two of five people believe that men make better business executives than women do. Gender biases are pronounced in both low and high Human Development Index (HDI) countries. These biases hold across regions, income, level of development and cultures—making them a global issue*" [8, 11].

Independently from the acting level, unconscious biases permeate our society and create inequity in various aspects of our lives like healthcare, employment, criminal justice, and education [12, 13]. Nowadays, social media also amplifies this phenomenon. It is well known that biases not only create political polarization but, based on the idea that "*similarity breeds connection*" may lead to homophily, which tends to homogenize people's networks in terms of sociodemographic, behavioral, and intrapersonal characteristics [14, 15]. Homophily favors perception bias and may, in turn, cause the development and/or persistence of implicit biases.

Hospitals and institutions are interested in reducing implicit biases, and interventions and training sessions are proposed in numerous settings (e.g., implicit bias training as police use-of-force reform) [13, 16, 17]. Interventions must be based on empirical tests and models to avoid increased biases due to ineffective training [13]. For instance, regarding assessment tools, the implicit association test (IAT) is the most common method to measure biases in research [9, 13, 18]. Regarding models of interventions, from the systematic review of Fitzgerald et al., it emerged that interventions requiring the engagement with other's perspectives are not successful in short-term implicit bias reduction. At the same time, the exposure to counterstereotypical exemplars provides better results [13].

13.2 Dimensions and Impact of Unconscious Bias in Healthcare

13.2.1 Patients' Perspective

Given for granted that doctors should always work following the Hippocratic Oath, the unconscious bias in medicine is still pervasive and may have a multifaceted and multilevel impact, not only influencing the patient–healthcare provider relationship but also reducing the diversity of medical personnel and directing the distribution of funding, resources, and career opportunities [1, 8]. Nevertheless, compared to other fields, such as the world of business, where it is commonly addressed, implicit bias is rarely covered in medicine [9].

Regarding the relationship between healthcare providers and patients, for example, the former may express implicit biases against marginalized groups of individuals, including minorities and disabled persons, even with consequences on medical decision-making [19]. Nevertheless, a proper response can be challenging for those witnessing these types of events since it would imply reporting a lack of professionalism of the physicians involved [8].

In terms of gender bias in medicine, as stated by Caroline Criado Perez in the book *Invisible Women*, evidence of discrimination against female patients can be found already in ancient Greek culture, although very progressive in many other aspects. Indeed, Aristotle considered *female nature a mutilated male nature* [20, 21]. Even if, fortunately, significant changes in medical evidence have occurred since then, much still has to be done and improved. Gender bias in medicine, as highlighted by Verdonk and colleagues, can be expressed in different forms like gender blindness (i.e., not taking it into account when it could be relevant), male bias (i.e., observer error rising from a predominantly male perspective and associated ways of thinking), gender role ideology (i.e., gender-influenced patients and healthcare providers attitude), and gender inequality [22].

All medical decisions are made on the basis of evidence demonstrated by research. Unfortunately, it became clear that for a long time, most medical research has been gender-biased, and this has had clinical consequences. For instance, Vitale and colleagues recently addressed how the elderly and women are under-represented in clinical trials investigating the effect of drugs on cardiovascular diseases [23]. Such attitude certainly hampers the knowledge of the efficacy of drugs on women and their potential different side effects. This lack of research cannot be acceptable anymore, considering that it is widely recognized that there are differences in pharmacokinetics and pharmacodynamics between women and men, which also play a significant role in drug metabolism [24]. As further evidence of the impact of such bias in this field, the "Yentl Syndrome" can be recalled. It refers to the short story "Yentl the Yeshiva Boy" written by Isaac Bashevis Singer and published for the first time in Yiddish in 1962, describing the story of an Ashkenazi Jewish woman in

Poland who took a male identity to study the Talmud law [25]. This reference was used by Bernardine Healy in 2001 to highlight that women could reach equality just if they were like men and, in particular, how this affects their assessment and treatment for cardiovascular diseases [26, 27]. In fact, in wealthier regions, the annual mortality rate from ischemic heart disease is higher for women compared to men due to underdiagnosis and undertreatment [26, 27]. Two studies published in 2011 on large cohorts (12,200 and 6558 women and men, respectively, in Sweden and Canada) demonstrated undertreatment of women with both drugs and procedures such as angiography than men [28, 29].

Similar to what has been described above for the cardiovascular field, this has been addressed by Curno et al. for HIV. Indeed, they demonstrated that women are underrepresented in research on HIV, even though it is well-known that in HIV, as for other diseases, sex and gender significantly influence factors such as the risk of acquisition and the rate of disease progression [24]. For instance, women, despite higher CD4 counts and lower viral loads at disease onset, may experience faster disease progression than men [24, 30, 31].

Therefore, even if it is well known that there are sex and gender differences in the prevalence, incidence, clinical manifestations, progression, or outcome of many diseases, still, much has to be done to include women in clinical trials and fill the gender gap. Willing to reduce this data gap, in 1991, the NIH launched the "Women's Health Initiative," a series of clinical studies aiming to improve health by addressing issues causing morbidity and mortality in postmenopausal women [26, 32]. Further, in 1993, the National Institution of Health Revitalization Act required that clinical trials include women and minorities [33]. In Canada, the Health Portfolio Sex-and Gender-Based Analysis (SGBA) Plus policy became effective in 2009 to promote inclusive research [34]. In 2016, the Sex and Gender Equity in Research (SAGER) guidelines were published to promote reporting sex and gender information in the research framework, data examination, results assessment, and understanding [35]. In line with these changes, scientific journals are revising their guidelines and policies [36]. For example, during the workshop "Sex-specific Reporting of Scientific Research" held by the US Institute of Medicine in 2011, several critical topics that editors and journals need to tackle to improve the gender-sensitive presentation of research, such as the importance of conducting sex-specific data analyses, were discussed [35].

Similarly, already in 2010, the US Institute of Medicine recommended that the International Committee of Medical Journal Editors (ICMJE) and other editors check for the inclusion of gender-disaggregated data in research papers reporting results of clinical trials [35].

Certainly all these norms are increasing awareness about gender implicit bias in medicine and are expected to reduce it in the near future. However, the persistence of biases also depends on the approach applied during medical education, where there is still a lack of proper training curricula [22]. For instance, Henrich et al., collecting data from the Association of American Medical Colleges' Curriculum Management and Information Tool (CurrMIT), demonstrated that only a few schools offered gender-related information in their curricula and/or had women's health courses [37]. Similar evidence was collected by Song and colleagues, who, in addition to assessing the presence of such classes in the curricula, trained six students to audit the first 2 years of the medical school curriculum for sex and gender-based course content in their institution. The audit revealed that most material was based on physiological and anatomical sex differences, not focusing on potential gender-based variability in diagnosis, prognosis, treatment, and outcomes [38]. Therefore, much still has to be done regarding the quantity and quality of gender education in medicine.

We should also consider that gender biases can be associated with ethnicity and age biases. For example, racial and ethnic disparities emerged in hospital readmission rates [39]. Higher rates of readmission have been reported in Black and Hispanic than in white patients for various diseases such as diabetes, heart failure, and acute myocardial infarction [39–43]. Aseltine and colleagues investigated these disparities in readmissions associated with women's reproductive health [39]. Analyzing a cohort of 167,857 patients admitted for vaginal delivery without complication and 75,552 patients admitted for cesarean delivery without complication from 2005 to 2012 demonstrated that 30-day readmission rates per 1000 patients were significantly higher among Black and Hispanic women after both cesarean and vaginal delivery [39]. Even if it might be easy to attribute such disparity to the hospital performance, as highlighted by the authors, it depends on a lack of community resources, such as the availability of general practitioners [39]. Moreover, in observing these results, the importance of genetic and biological factors and racial predispositions should be addressed. In fact, it is well known that in Black mothers and fetuses, there is a higher prevalence of genetic predisposition to inflammation, which may cause postpartum endometritis and, therefore, hospital readmission [39, 44, 45]. Given this, tailored postpartum programs should be developed to provide the best care and prevent readmission and potential complications.

Chambers and colleagues addressed racism in maternal health from a different point of view, proposing a clinicians' perspective [46]. The authors administered 25 semi-structured interviews to perinatal care clinicians practicing in the San Francisco Bay Area and serving women of various races [46]. Three main themes emerged from this research: (i) *provision of inequitable care* due to racism influencing clinicians' racist stereotypes and credences; (ii) *surveillance of Black women and families*, punitive care, and treatment; and (iii) *structural care issues*, it encompasses both past and present repercussions of racially biased healthcare practices in gynecology [46]. In line with the need to dismantle such radicated and structural behavior and all the consequent biased conduct, in 2019, California passed the Dignity in Pregnancy and Childbirth Act (SB 464) [47]. More initiatives and laws of these types should be implemented in the near future to guarantee full equity in patients' treatment.

Considering the overall racism in healthcare, Black women have higher incidence and mortality rates of cervical cancer than white women, and they are often diagnosed at the end stages [48–50]. This is undoubtedly related to the fact that Black women have less access to screening programs. In fact, as for other types of cancer, such as cervical tumors, screening is essential to reach an early diagnosis.

Strategies like the "Face your Health" program, an outreach educational initiative encouraging African Americans to be screened for this type of cancer, will undoubtedly improve such rates [51].

Recently, Washington et al., using the Discrimination in Medical Settings scale (DMS) as part of a pilot mobile health (mHealth) cervical cancer intervention study, evaluated the occurrence of discrimination in medical settings for Black women. In a sample of 48 patients, 23 reported being treated with less courtesy, and as many reported receiving poorer service [48]. Overall, Black women experienced high levels of perceived discrimination [48].

The recent COVID-19 pandemic has emphasized the disparities in healthcare. In the United States, disease prevalence and death rates were higher among Blacks, Hispanics, and Asian Americans, with three times higher hospitalization rates in Native Americans and Alaska natives than white patients [52]. Moreover, socioeconomic status, gender, age, and education played an additional role with a significant negative impact [52]. A study on 21 Latinx immigrant women in New York City during the pandemic and their perception of racism and xenophobia in their healthcare experiences showed that they faced discrimination at different levels. They reported enduring systemic inequalities in social and economic realms, along with personal experiences of biased medical treatment and fears of being victimized by social institutions [52].

Similarly, the European Institute for Gender Equality described how the pandemic aggravated healthcare inequality and revealed how *gender intersects with occupation, age, and migration status to increase vulnerability to infection* [53]. Indeed, the SARS-COV2 outbreak caused a massive shift to remote working, but this option, which guaranteed more protection, was not accessible to all workers [53]. According to Eurostat data, it then emerged that most women are part of the so-called essential workers, accounting *for 88% of personal care workers, 84% of cleaners and helpers, 73% of education workers, and 72% of health professionals in EU countries* [53]. Workers on the frontline were obviously at higher risk of interacting with infected people and, therefore, getting sick. In various European Countries like Germany, Italy, and Spain, around 70% of infections among health workers occurred in women [54–57]. Migrant female workers of working age who are highly involved in care and domestic jobs were mainly exposed to COVID-19 infection [53].

During the COVID-19 pandemic, also ageism emerged worldwide [58]. For instance, France failed to report mortality rates of the elderly in nursing homes as if they were valued less [59]. Some countries have applied stricter restrictions on older adults, increasing their sense of isolation and social media via initiatives like the hashtag "#BoomerRemover" have negatively influenced the perception of COVID-19 giving a distorted message to society [58]. Indeed, due to this, the mortality rates of older adults were justified and perceived as inevitable, while younger adults believed to be invulnerable [58].

Unfortunately, implicit biases toward age affect healthcare beyond the recent pandemic. The term ageism, coined by Dr. Robert Butler in 1968, accurately describes the prejudice of one age group against another, stemming from stereotypes and discrimination [60]. In healthcare, such discriminatory behavior can lead to delayed diagnoses, inappropriate care, and low quality of life [60]. For instance, as previously mentioned, Vitale and colleagues highlighted the exclusion of not only women but also the elderly from clinical trials [23].

Moreover, it is well known that older patients with HIV may face additional challenges [61]. In fact, despite the therapeutic improvements for this disease, the elderly often do not benefit from such achievements because of a late diagnosis (CD4 count below 350 cells per cubic millimeter, or with an AIDS-defining event, regardless of the CD4 cell count) [62–64]. According to The UK Health Security Agency report: *HIV testing, PrEP, new HIV diagnoses and care outcomes for people accessing HIV services: 2024 report,* the rate of late diagnosis increased by 3% from 2022 to 2023 with *the highest proportions of late diagnoses among people aged 50 years and over* (*55% for those aged 65 years and over*) [64]. Further, *the increase in the number of late diagnoses since 2022 is largely among people of black ethnicity (40% increase from 259 to 362).* This might be seen with an *intersectional perspective* [61]. In fact, individuals may experience various types of discrimination, for instance, gender, age, disease, and race-related [61]. In line with this, Garcia-Pena et al. highlighted how, in Mexico, senior individuals with diverse sexual orientation and gender identities are often unseen and their needs unmet [61]. They face more impediments in social service and healthcare, resulting in worse physical and mental health status. The study of Fredriksen-Goldsen et al. using population-based data from the Washington State Behavioral Risk Factor Surveillance System demonstrated that there are health disparities between sexually diverse and straight people [65].

The results of a survey conducted in 2017 by the Center for American Progress showed that 6–9% of lesbian, gay, bisexual, or queer patients report difficulties with healthcare providers, including discriminatory language, lack of acknowledgment of family members, and denial of care [66]. Percentages rise to 29% for transgender patients [66]. Such behaviors discourage access to care. Similarly, in January 2016, the first report on transgender equality by the British Women and Equalities Committee demonstrated that transgender patients still face prejudice and a lack of understanding. Indeed, according to the report, "*GPs too often lack understanding, and in some cases, this leads to appropriate care not being provided*" [67]. Discrimination may occur in various forms, such as misgendering (using the correct pronoun), deadnaming (using the previous first name that typically reflects the gender assigned at birth), and objectification (being treated as an object of transsexuality) [68]. Discrimination and ignorance among healthcare professionals may lead to postponing or even refusing medical care [68]. Interestingly, an interview study revealed that transgender individuals experienced discrimination in their access to care, even from so-called trans-specialists (specialists who should support them during the medical transition). Further research by the same researchers demonstrated that, among other factors, specific challenges related to the validation of the diagnosis of transsexuality, as well as uncertainties regarding its classification as a mental illness, induce discriminatory behaviors [68]. This shows that much work remains to be done to properly educate and train physicians to provide a safe, bias-free healthcare environment for all patients.

13.2.2 Healthcare Providers' Perspective

So far, we have addressed implicit biases toward patients, but they might also be toward healthcare providers and colleagues. A survey of 6512 US physicians showed that 21.6% experienced care refusal from patients or caregivers because of physicians' attributes at least once in the previous year [69]. Moreover, especially female physicians and ethnic and racial minority physicians were victims of discrimination and mistreatment perpetrated by patients, family members, and visitors [69]. This was independently associated with higher odds of burnout. Specialists in emergency medicine were at higher risk of mistreatment than physicians practicing pathology or radiology, given the less contact with patients of the latter [69].

Similar trends emerged in the study of Kauff and colleagues in Germany [70]. Indeed, collecting the evaluations of more than 140,000 physicians on Jameda (i.e., a German platform where patients rate physicians) demonstrated that general practitioners with a migration background and female physicians received worse ratings [70]. As shown by the study of Templeton et al., discrimination against women persists throughout their careers without disappearing with age or seniority [71]. Moreover, even if empathy has been linked to improved health outcomes, such as patient satisfaction and treatment adherence, according to the literature, empathy is influenced by gender, and it seems to be perceived differently by patients if expressed by male or female physicians [72, 73]. Indeed, female physicians are rated positively if they behave in line with expected gender roles, such as using a softer voice and having less dominance. In contrast, for male physicians, higher satisfaction was associated with a broader range of behaviors only partly related to typical gender roles [74].

Interestingly, gender bias is contradicted by daily clinical practice. Indeed, as demonstrated in a recent study, patients had lower mortality and readmission rates when treated by female physicians [75]. The proper divulgation of such evidence to patients and healthcare staff should be promoted to dismantle the prejudices and biases that female physicians still encounter.

Regarding gender, a recent survey involving 24 transgender and/or gender-expansive physicians revealed that they still face both overt and subtle biases related to their identity and gender presentation [76]. The participants reported experiencing emotional distress due to various factors, including transphobia, isolation, and misgendering [76]. They mentioned the ongoing stigma from colleagues, a lack of representation in medicine and the community, and a poor understanding of nonbinary gender identities among colleagues and patients [76]. As demonstrated in the literature, increasing contact with LGBTQIA+ individuals could help prevent implicit bias and mitigate all the negative consequences previously mentioned [76, 77].

Considering race and the previously mentioned racial biases toward patients, several studies have described implicit prejudices among physicians against Black, Hispanic, American Indian, and other colleagues with darker skin tones, highlighting significant social impacts [78]. For instance, as noted in the commentary by Fernandez et al., the number of Hispanic physicians in the United States has progressively decreased in recent decades, resulting in overall underrepresentation in medicine and a further leak in the pipeline within the medical academic environment. Indeed, Hispanic physicians make up only 6% of the full-time staff and 3% of the full professors [79]. Ethnoracism and implicit biases undoubtedly contribute to this phenomenon. In fact, Hispanic medical students often feel unrecognized and isolated, fighting against stereotypes such as the perception that having a Spanish accent indicates low competence and education [80].

The results of a recent survey conducted in the Canadian province of Ontario, including 46 physicians and trainees who identified as Black (African/Afro-Canadian/African American/Afro-Caribbean), demonstrate the occurrence of harmful discrimination from peers, patients, and superiors and highlight the importance and need for tailored mentorship and educational programs on discrimination and bias [81]. As highlighted in a systematic review about discrimination toward physicians of color, racial bias strongly impacts not only individuals but also the system [82]. It leads to job dissatisfaction and intentions to leave, and discrimination is associated with adverse health outcomes [82]. It is also very important to underline the role of healthcare organizations since, so far, they seem to have tolerated biased and discriminatory behaviors of patients according to physicians' characteristics such as gender, ethnicity, and race [82]. Certainly, healthcare organizations are expected to develop policies and programs supporting diverse physicians from discrimination.

13.2.3 Implicit Bias in Physicians' Recruitment and Career

Implicit biases also influence the recruitment of physicians and their professional advancement. It is well known that, even though women have recently outnumbered men among medical school graduates, they remain underrepresented in leadership roles within the medical field, particularly in academia [83–85]. For instance, in the United States, women comprise only 25% of full professors and 18% of Department Chairs [84]. Likewise, evidence gathered from five hospitals in Lombardia, Italy, shows that women earn 18% less than men and encounter more obstacles in progressing from low to mid-level positions due to a "sticky floor" effect, which inhibits career advancement for women [86].

As nicely described by Hui and colleagues, gender biases significantly contribute to these disparities, but they are difficult to dismantle because they are underrecognized, not consciously perceived, and because they persist throughout medical professional's career [85].

Various strategies should be systematically implemented for candidate selection and hiring, from using inclusive language in job postings to proper bias training for search committees [87]. This approach generally applies not only to gender bias but also to any other potential implicit biases. A robust education in diversity, equity, and inclusivity (DEI) should ensure the selection of the best candidate, free from any bias [87]. Moreover, institutions should create a supportive environment that provides career flexibility, guarantees maternal and paternal leave, and establishes mentorship and sponsorship programs [87].

A recent study based on the assessment of 101 named and anonymous applications for a training program for junior doctors demonstrated that anonymization increased the proportion of successful female candidates from 27% to 46% [84]. Similarly, research analyzing data on applications from 1995 to 2018 to the Leiden University International Study Fund (LISF) revealed that the number of grant applications of women and men was equal. Still, women had lower success despite the equivalent quality of the applications when assessed anonymously [88].

Biases hinder the selection and careers not just of women but also of all minorities, particularly in certain specialties. For instance, in 2017, underrepresented minorities comprised only 13% of emergency residents [89]. There is a significant lack of medical school applications from Black students [90]. This is undoubtedly due to limited access to information about career options, financial barriers, as well as biases and stereotypes that obstruct opportunities for minorities entering medicine [90]. Creating a diverse healthcare workforce is crucial for providing high-quality medical care. Embracing diversity can improve healthcare accessibility for marginalized groups, engage a broader range of participants in developing effective care policies, and lead to more innovative research on the factors contributing to health inequities [90].

13.3 The Unconscious Bias in Diagnostic Imaging

Also, radiology is highly affected by implicit bias as expressed by the low percentage of "underrepresented in medicine" (racial and ethnic populations that are underrepresented in the medical profession relative to their numbers in the general population) in this specialty and especially in interventional [91].

In line with this, Chapman and colleagues also demonstrated the underrepresentation of women in imaging. As reported by Seely, gender disparities within organizations create obstacles for women in radiology, significantly hindering their advancement into leadership roles, concepts also confirmed in a recent systematic review [92–94]. An interesting study reviewing the residency letters of recommendation for 736 diagnostic radiology residency applicants to Duke University from the 2015 to 2016 interview season applied the psychological framework of agency and communality, which describes masculine and feminine domains in Western society [95]. Using this method, the authors showed that the variation in the use of agentic and communal language in the letters is influenced by the demographics of both the applicants and the writers [95]. More agentic descriptors were used for white and Asian applicants compared to Black and Latinx applicants, confirming the favorable biases toward white candidates previously discussed [95]. Junior faculty members employed communal and agentic terms [95].

Thus, tailored programs should promote inclusion and diverse mentorship, and courses in inclusive writing should be promoted in radiology departments.

13.3.1 Unconscious Bias and Artificial Intelligence (AI)

Artificial intelligence sees one of its primary fields of application in medical imaging. Despite the remarkable achievements of machine learning and AI modeling, these technologies may suffer from biases. Recent studies have shown that cutting-edge models can reinforce racial and gender biases, as demonstrated by their tendency to generate images of white men for requests like "CEO portraits," while depicting minority women for requests such as "social worker portraits" and individuals from racial minorities for "forensic sketches of possible suspects" [96].

Models can generate predictions about sensitive factors, such as patients' race, age, gender, and ethnicity, which are assumed to have been stripped of identifying information prior to the development of the model [96]. Recent research indicates that AI technologies can utilize latent information in chest X-rays to forecast sensitive characteristics. However, the specific elements contributing to these predictions are often unknown to users [96]. While some features, like the role of the sternum and upper ribs, may contribute to the development of these models, there remains a lack of clarity in identifying features that consistently influence the prediction of sensitive attributes. Consequently, these sensitive characteristics could affect final model outcomes, exacerbating existing clinical biases linked to specific medical issues or datasets, often without the end user's knowledge. Similarly, through the analysis of radiographs, models might extract demographic details, essential health metrics (such as body mass index), and indicators of chronic conditions (including cardiomegaly, vascular calcifications, and osteopenia) to predict the costs associated with care. An AI approach that leverages this information could potentially aid in developing methods to reduce unnecessary healthcare spending; however, malicious parties could use similar frameworks based on sensitive factors to deny care to those at higher risk [96–99].

Indeed, since AI is built on data from *human-made datasets,* many of the implicit biases discussed in this chapter can be transferred to AI models [100]. For instance, Bachina et al. conducted a retrospective review of chest X-ray images from two publicly available datasets, MIMIC-CXR and CheXpert, which identified underdiagnosis rates linked to different racial and ethnic labels, particularly for Black, Hispanic/Latino, and Asian individuals compared to white individuals [100, 101]. The consequences of underdiagnosing diseases in entire racial or ethnic groups can be significant, resulting in delayed care and poor outcomes [100]. Furthermore, excluding specific demographics and subsets of patients may lead to their under-representation in AI models and biased training datasets, exacerbating existing biases. The concept of automation bias involves preference for machine-generated recommendations, even in light of contradictory evidence, thereby relinquishing decision-making responsibility to automated technology [96]. In radiology, this can result in significant interpretation errors, manifesting as omission or commission errors [96].

In line with this, Curto and colleagues, who investigated potential biases against the poor in Natural Language Processing word vectors such as Google Word2Vec, Twitter, and Wikipedia GloVe, demonstrated that the bias in Google Word2Vec was more pronounced for belief-related terms. In contrast, Twitter GloVe showed increased bias concerning terms that pertain to behavior [102].

Automation bias in radiology is more likely to affect patients with lower socio-economic status and/or systems with lower resources. Systems that lack sufficient resources or expert personnel, especially those with a shortage of radiologists skilled in AI, tend to depend heavily on AI technologies due to the high demand for services and the growing complexity of medical studies [96].

Therefore, effort must be devoted to reducing AI automation bias, ensuring that AI systems are representative of minorities and are built with fairness, without data distribution shifts.

13.4 Strategies to Mitigate Unconscious Bias and Future Perspectives

Since it is challenging to recognize implicit bias and we can all be affected, awareness is the first step to reducing its consequences. According to Schiavo, we should apply strategies to reduce implicit biases. For instance, we should regularly check and challenge our own biases, act with empathy and compassion, identify behaviors that may contribute to biases, and engage in strategies to mitigate them [8].

Over time, several tools have also been proposed. For instance, the *Harvard implicit association test* (https://implicit.harvard.edu/implicit/takeatest.html) assesses opinions and convictions that individuals might hesitate to disclose or find difficult to express [18].

Moreover, as stated above, the recruitment policies and strategies favoring DEI should be systematically implemented for candidate selection and hiring, from using inclusive language in job postings to proper bias training for search committees.

As described above, significant progress has been made to mitigate the negative impact of unconscious bias in healthcare over the past few decades, yet much work remains. Current political trends aimed at diminishing civil rights, diversity, and inclusion while advancing racism, are spreading and pose unprecedented threats to democracy that cannot be overlooked. For example, in the United States, the directive to federal agencies to eliminate "radical and wasteful Diversity, Equity, and Inclusion programs" and to remove websites and public platforms "promoting gender ideology" risks diminishing the value of individual merit and commitment in selecting individuals for essential jobs in this field and could hinder scientific advancements in medicine [103]. Unfortunately, scientific societies have begun to alter or cancel their DEI programs and are abandoning DEI-focused language and initiatives [104, 105]. Furthermore, many scientists find their research jeopardized simply because it addresses gender and racial issues. This is evident in a project regarding the sexual orientation and gender identity of cancer patients, which has already yielded significant results, but will be scrapped under a new executive order [106]. In this incredibly challenging and difficult historical moment, scientific communities should uphold their principles and maintain their educational and moral commitment to all citizens and minorities. For instance, the American Society of Naturalists has communicated to its members that it will continue "supporting and promoting diversity not only as a goal but as a fundamental value" [104]. We advocate for further initiatives like the SystemicDisease.com website launched by Jessica Cerdena and Tehreem Rehman, which fosters understanding of prejudice in healthcare while creating a virtual community that supports and advocates for those who have faced discrimination [107].

13.5 Conclusions

In conclusion, implicit bias has a significant negative impact in the medical field, acting at different levels and in various contexts, influencing not only the patient–healthcare relationship and the overall access to care but also affecting the clinical and academic career and the collegial relationship among healthcare providers. The scientific and academic communities should defend the important achievements of the last decades, which helped reduce some biases, and work hard to dismantle those still existing, aiming to improve the quality of care for everybody.

References

1. Sabin JA. Tackling implicit bias in health care. N Engl J Med. 2022;387:105–7. https://doi.org/10.1056/NEJMp2201180.
2. Understanding Bias: A resource guide. https://www.justice.gov/d9/fieldable-panel-panes/basic-panes/attachments/2021/09/29/understanding_bias_content.pdf. Accessed on 18 Dec 2024.
3. Implicit Bias. American Psychological Association. https://www.apa.org/topics/implicit-bias. Accessed on 18 Dec 2024.
4. Greenwald AG, Banaji MR. Implicit social cognition: attitudes, self-esteem, and stereotypes. Psychol Rev. 1995;102:4–27.
5. Greenwald AG, Lai CK. Implicit social cognition. Annu Rev Psychol. 2020;71:419–45. https://doi.org/10.1146/annurev-psych-010419-050837.
6. Storm K, Reiss LK, Guenther EA, Clar-Novak M, Muhr SL. Unconscious bias in the HRM literature: towards a critical-reflexive approach. Hum Resour Manag Rev. 2023;33:100969. https://doi.org/10.1016/j.hrmr.2023.100969.
7. Roberson L, Block CJ. Racioethnicity and job performance: a review and critique of theoretical perspectives on the causes of group differences. Res Organ Behav. 2001;23:247–325.
8. Schiavo R. Challenging implicit bias: a call for action. J Commun Healthc. 2024;17:311–3. https://doi.org/10.1080/17538068.2024.2432170.
9. Gopal DP, Chetty U, O'Donnell P, Gajria C, Blackadder-Weinstein J. Implicit bias in healthcare: clinical practice, research and decision making. Future Healthc J. 2021;8:40–8. https://doi.org/10.7861/fhj.2020-0233.
10. Payne BK, Vuletich HA, Brown-Iannuzzi JL. Historical roots of implicit bias in slavery. Proc Natl Acad Sci USA. 2019;116:11693–8. https://doi.org/10.1073/pnas.1818816116.
11. 2023 Gender Social Norms Index (GSNI). Breaking down gender biases: Shifting social norms towards gender equality. Human Development Resources https://hdr.undp.org/content/2023-gender-social-norms-index-gsni#/indicies/GSNI. Accessed on 23 Dec 2024.

12. Stier AJ, Sajjadi S, Karimi F, Bettencourt LMA, Berman MG. Implicit racial biases are lower in more populous more diverse and less segregated US cities. Nat Commun. 2024;15:961. https://doi.org/10.1038/s41467-024-45013-8.
13. Fitzgerald C, Martin A, Berner D, Hurst S. Interventions designed to reduce implicit prejudices and implicit stereotypes in real world contexts: a systematic review. BMC Psychol. 2019;7:29. https://doi.org/10.1186/s40359-019-0299-7.
14. Modgil S, Singh RK, Gupta S, Dennehy D. A confirmation bias view on social media induced polarisation during Covid-19. Inf Syst Front. 2021;20:1–25. https://doi.org/10.1007/s10796-021-10222-9.
15. McPherson M, Smith-Lovin L, Cook JM. Birds of a feather: homophily in social networks. Annu Rev Sociol. 2001;27:415–44.
16. Machado MA, Lugo AM. A behavioral analysis of two strategies to eliminate racial bias in police use of force. Behav Anal Pract. 2021;15:1221–31. https://doi.org/10.1007/s40617-021-00551-1.
17. Boscardin CK. Reducing implicit bias through curricular interventions. J Gen Intern Med. 2015;30:1726–8. https://doi.org/10.1007/s11606-015-3496-y.
18. Implicit Association Test. Harvard University Office for equity, diversity, inclusion and belonging. https://edib.harvard.edu/implicit-association-test-iat#:~:text=The%20Implicit%20Association%20Test%20(IAT,you%20did%20not%20know%20about. Accessed on 23 Dec 2024.
19. Vela MB, Erondu AI, Smith NA, Peek ME, Woodruff JN, Chin MH. Eliminating explicit and implicit biases in health care: evidence and research needs. Annu Rev Public Health. 2022;43:477–501. https://doi.org/10.1146/annurev-publhealth-052620-103528.
20. Perez CC. Invisible women. Exposing data bias in a world designed for men. Part IV: going to the doctor. London: Vintage; 2020. p. 193–236.
21. Bonnard JB. Male and female bodies according to ancient Greek physicians. Clio. Online. 2013. http://journals.openedition.org/cliowgh/339;;37 https://doi.org/10.4000/cliowgh.339.
22. Verdonk P, Benschop YW, de Haes HC, Lagro-Janssen TL. From gender bias to gender awareness in medical education. Adv Health Sci Educ Theory Pract. 2009;14:135–52. https://doi.org/10.1007/s10459-008-9100-z.
23. Vitale C, Fini M, Spoletini I, Lainscak M, Seferovic P, Rosano GM. Under-representation of elderly and women in clinical trials. Int J Cardiol. 2017;232:216–21. https://doi.org/10.1016/j.ijcard.2017.01.018.
24. Curno MJ, Rossi S, Hodges-Mameletzis I, Johnston R, Price MA, Heidari S. A systematic review of the inclusion (or exclusion) of women in HIV research: from clinical studies of antiretrovirals and vaccines to cure strategies. J Acquir Immune Defic Syndr. 2016;71:181–8. https://doi.org/10.1097/QAI.0000000000000842.
25. Isaac Bashevis Singer. Yentl and the Yashiva Boy. Publisher: Farrar, Straus and Giroux, New York; Publication Date: 1983; ISBN 10: 0374293473
26. Healy B. The Yentl syndrome. N Engl J Med. 1991;325:274–6. https://doi.org/10.1056/NEJM199107253250408.
27. Merz CN. The Yentl syndrome is alive and well. Eur Heart J. 2011;32:1313–5. https://doi.org/10.1093/eurheartj/ehr083.
28. Johnston N, Schenck-Gustafsson K, Lagerqvist B. Are we using cardiovascular medications and coronary angiography appropriately in men and women with chest pain? Eur Heart J. 2011;32:1331–6. https://doi.org/10.1093/eurheartj/ehr009.
29. Bugiardini R, Yan AT, Yan RT, Fitchett D, Langer A, Manfrini O, Goodman SG. Factors influencing underutilization of evidence-based therapies in women on behalf of the Canadian Acute Coronary Syndrome Registry I and II Investigators. Eur Heart J. 2011;32:1337–44. https://doi.org/10.1093/eurheartj/ehr027.
30. Gandhi M, Bacchetti P, Miotti P, et al. Does patient sex affect human immunodeficiency virus levels? Clin Infect Dis. 2002;35:313–22.
31. Jarrin I, Geskus R, Bhaskaran K, et al. Gender differences in HIV progression to AIDS and death in industrialized countries: slower disease progression following HIV seroconversion in women. Am J Epidemiol. 2008;168:532–40.

32. Women's Health Initiative. Changing the future of women's health. A landmark study since 1992. https://www.whi.org/. Accessed on 29 Dec 2024.
33. Nichols FH. History of the women's health movement in the 20th century. J Obstet Gynecol Neonatal Nurs. 2000;29:56–64. https://doi.org/10.1111/j.1552-6909.2000.tb02756.x.
34. Health Portfolio Sex- and Gender-Based Analysis Plus Policy: Advancing Equity, Diversity and Inclusion. Government of Canada. https://www.canada.ca/en/health-canada/corporate/transparency/heath-portfolio-sex-gender-based-analysis-policy.html. Accessed on 28 Dec 2024.
35. Heidari S, Babor TF, Castro P, Tort S, Curno M. Equidade de sexo e gênero na pesquisa: fundamentação das diretrizes SAGER e uso recomendado [Sex and Gender Equity in Research: rationale for the SAGER guidelines and recommended use]. Epidemiol Serv Saude. 2017;26:665–75.
36. Lee H, Pak YK, Yeo EJ, Kim YS, Paik HY, Lee SK. It is time to integrate sex as a variable in preclinical and clinical studies. Exp Mol Med. 2018;50:1–2. https://doi.org/10.1038/s12276-018-0122-1.
37. Henrich JB, Viscoli CM. What do medical schools teach about women's health and gender differences? Acad Med. 2006;81:476–82. https://doi.org/10.1097/01.ACM.0000222268.60211.fc.
38. Song MM, Jones BG, Casanova RA. Auditing sex- and gender-based medicine (SGBM) content in medical school curriculum: a student scholar model. Biol Sex Differ. 2016;7:40. https://doi.org/10.1186/s13293-016-0102-x.
39. Aseltine RH Jr, Yan J, Fleischman S, Katz M, DeFrancesco M. Racial and ethnic disparities in hospital readmissions after delivery. Obstet Gynecol. 2015;126(5):1040–7. https://doi.org/10.1097/AOG.0000000000001090.
40. Kim H, Ross JS, Melkus GD, Zhao Z, Boockvar K. Scheduled and unscheduled hospital readmissions among patients with diabetes. Am J Manag Care. 2010;16:760–7.
41. Joynt KE, Orav EJ, Jha AK. Thirty-day readmission rates for Medicare beneficiaries by race and site of care. JAMA. 2011;305:675–81.
42. Alexander M, Grumbach K, Remy L, Rowell R, Massie BM. Congestive heart failure hospitalizations and survival in California: patterns according to race/ethnicity. Am Heart J. 1999;137:919–27.
43. Rodriguez F, Joynt KE, López L, Saldaña F, Jha AK. Readmission rates for Hispanic Medicare beneficiaries with heart failure and acute myocardial infarction. Am Heart J. 2011;162:254–61.
44. Anum EA, Springel EH, Shriver MD, Strauss JF 3rd. Genetic contributions to disparities in preterm birth. Pediatr Res. 2009;65:1–9.
45. Menon R, Pearce B, Velez DR, Merialdi M, Williams SM, Fortunato SJ, et al. Racial disparity in pathophysiologic pathways of preterm birth based on genetic variants. Reprod Biol Endocrinol. 2009;7:62.
46. Chambers BD, Taylor B, Nelson T, Harrison J, Bell A, O'Leary A, Arega HA, Hashemi S, McKenzie-Sampson S, Scott KA, Raine-Bennett T, Jackson AV, Kuppermann M, McLemore MR. Clinicians' perspectives on racism and black women's maternal health. Womens Health Rep (New Rochelle). 2022;3:476–82. https://doi.org/10.1089/whr.2021.0148.
47. SB-464 California Dignity in Pregnancy and Childbirth Act. Senate Bill No. 464 Chapter 533 https://leginfo.legislature.ca.gov/faces/billTextClient.xhtml?bill_id=201920200SB464. Accessed on 28 Dec 2024.
48. Washington A, Randall J. "We're not taken seriously": describing the experiences of perceived discrimination in medical settings for black Women. J Racial Ethn Health Disparities. 2023;10:883–91. https://doi.org/10.1007/s40615-022-01276-9.
49. Yoo W, Kim S, Huh WK, Dilley S, Coughlin SS, Partridge EE, et al. Recent trends in racial and regional disparities in cervical cancer incidence and mortality in United States. PLoS One. 2017;12(2):e0172548.
50. Siegel RL, Miller KD, Fuchs HE, Jemal A. Cancer statistics, 2021. CA Cancer J Clin. 2021;71:7–33.
51. Face Your Health Program. U.S. Centers for disease control and prevention. https://www.cdc.gov/cervical-cancer/face-your-health/index.html#:~:text=Face%20Your%20Health%20is%20an,get%20screened%20for%20cervical%20cancer. Accessed on 29 Dec 2024.

52. Mheidly N, Fares NY, Fares MY, Fares J. Emerging health disparities during the COVID-19 pandemic. Avicenna J Med. 2022;13:60–4. https://doi.org/10.1055/s-0042-1759842.
53. Gender Equality Index 2021: Health. European Institute for Gender Equality (EIGE) https://eige.europa.eu/publications-resources/toolkits-guides/gender-equality-index-2021-report/covid-19-pandemic-aggravates-and-brings-forth-health-inequalities?language_content_entity=en. Accessed on 29 Dec 2024.
54. Rozenberg S, Vandromme J, Martin C. Are we equal in adversity? Does Covid-19 affect women and men differently? Maturitas. 2020;138:62–8. https://doi.org/10.1016/j.maturitas.2020.05.009.
55. Hasell J, Mathieu E, Beltekian D, Macdonald B, Giattino C, Ortiz-Ospina E, Roser M, Ritchie H. A cross-country database of COVID-19 testing. Sci Data. 2020;7(1):345. https://doi.org/10.1038/s41597-020-00688-8.
56. Our world in data. Coronavirus (COVID-19) testing. https://ourworldindata.org/coronavirus-testing. Accessed on 29 Dec 2024.
57. Johns Hopkins University and Medicine. Coronavirus Research Center. https://coronavirus.jhu.edu/us-map. Accessed on 29 Dec 2024.
58. Fraser S, Lagacé M, Bongué B, Ndeye N, Guyot J, Bechard L, Garcia L, Taler V; CCNA Social Inclusion and Stigma Working Group; Adam S, Beaulieu M, Bergeron CD, Boudjemadi V, Desmette D, Donizzetti AR, Éthier S, Garon S, Gillis M, Levasseur M, Lortie-Lussier M, Marier P, Robitaille A, Sawchuk K, Lafontaine C, Tougas F. Ageism and COVID-19: what does our society's response say about us? Age Ageing. 2020;49:692–5. https://doi.org/10.1093/ageing/afaa097.
59. Boumedienne A. Coronavirus: Le Nombre de décès en Ehpad probablement beaucoup plus lourd que le bilan officiel. https://www.20minutes.fr/sante/2748183-20200325-coronavirus-nombre-deces-ephad-probablement-beaucoup-plus-lourd-bilan-officiel. Accessed on 29 Dec 2024.
60. González-García V, Chávez-García CL, Girón-Castillo JE, Reyes-Cedeño B, Sosa-Tinoco E. Combating ageism: awareness and best practices in healthcare for older people. Gac Med Mex. 2024;160:347–9. English. https://doi.org/10.24875/GMM.M24000903.
61. García-Peña C, Medina-Campos RH, Pérez-Zepeda MU, Vázquez-García J, Terán D, Torre-Rosas A. Forgotten older people: health system debt. Gac Med Mex. 2024;160:233–8. https://doi.org/10.24875/GMM.M24000894.
62. Mugavero MJ, Castellano C, Edelman D, Hicks C. Late diagnosis of HIV infection: the role of age and sex. Am J Med. 2007;120:370–3. https://doi.org/10.1016/j.amjmed.2006.05.050.
63. The Lancet Hiv. Time to tackle late diagnosis. Lancet HIV. 2022 Mar;9(3):e139. https://doi.org/10.1016/S2352-3018(22)00040-6.
64. HIV testing, PrEP, new HIV diagnoses and care outcomes for people accessing HIV services: 2024 report. UK health security agency. https://www.gov.uk/government/statistics/hiv-annual-data-tables/hiv-testing-prep-new-hiv-diagnoses-and-care-outcomes-for-people-accessing-hiv-services-2024-report#late-hiv-diagnosis-and-presentation. Accessed on 15 Jan 2025.
65. Fredriksen-Goldsen KI, Romanelli M, Jung HH, Kim HJ. Health, economic, and social disparities among lesbian, gay, bisexual, and sexually diverse adults: results from a population-based study. Behav Med. 2024;50:141–52. https://doi.org/10.1080/08964289.2022.2153787.
66. Franklin CC. Poorer health in the LGBTQ+ community due to fear of mistreatment. J Pediatric Orthopaedic Soc North Am. 2023:5(S1). https://doi.org/10.55275/JPOSNA-2023-625.
67. Wise J. Doctors are prejudiced against transgender patients, MPs say. BMJ. 2016;352:i252. https://doi.org/10.1136/bmj.i252.
68. Skuban-Eiseler T, Orzechowski M, Steger F. Discrimination experiences of transgender individuals in healthcare: an interview study on the perspective of health professionals specializing in the treatment of transgender individuals. Int J Equity Health. 2024;23:225. https://doi.org/10.1186/s12939-024-02313-1.
69. Dyrbye LN, West CP, Sinsky CA, Trockel M, Tutty M, Satele D, Carlasare L, Shanafelt T. Physicians' experiences with mistreatment and discrimination by patients, families, and

visitors and association with burnout. JAMA Netw Open. 2022;5:e2213080. https://doi.org/10.1001/jamanetworkopen.2022.13080.

70. Kauff M, Anslinger J, Christ O, Niemann M, Geierhos M, Huster L. Ethnic and gender-based prejudice towards medical doctors? The relationship between physicians' ethnicity, gender, and ratings on a physician rating website. J Soc Psychol. 2022;162:540–8. https://doi.org/10.1080/00224545.2021.1927944.
71. Templeton K, Bernstein C, Sukhera J, Nora LM, Newman C, Burstin H, Guille C, Lynn L, Schwarze ML, Sen S, Busis N. Gender-based differences in burnout: issues faced by women physicians. Washington, DC: NAM Perspectives. Discussion Paper, National Academy of Medicine; 2019. https://doi.org/10.31478/201905a.
72. Surchat C, Carrard V, Gaume J, Berney A, Clair C. Impact of physician empathy on patient outcomes: a gender analysis. Br J Gen Pract. 2022;72:e99–e107. https://doi.org/10.3399/BJGP.2021.0193.
73. Decety J, Fotopoulou A. Why empathy has a beneficial impact on others in medicine: unifying theories. Front Behav Neurosci. 2015;8:457. https://doi.org/10.3389/fnbeh.2014.00457.
74. Mast MS, Hall JA, Köckner C, Choi E. Physician gender affects how physician nonverbal behavior is related to patient satisfaction. Med Care. 2008;46(12):1212–8. https://doi.org/10.1097/MLR.0b013e31817e1877.
75. Miyawaki A, Jena AB, Rotenstein LS, Tsugawa Y. Comparison of hospital mortality and readmission rates by physician and patient sex. Ann Intern Med. 2024;177(5):598–608. https://doi.org/10.7326/M23-3163.
76. Westafer LM, Freiermuth CE, Lall MD, Muder SJ, Ragone EL, Jarman AF. Experiences of transgender and gender expansive physicians. JAMA Netw Open. 2022;5(6):e2219791. https://doi.org/10.1001/jamanetworkopen.2022.19791.
77. Wittlin NM, Dovidio JF, Burke SE, Przedworski JM, Herrin J, Dyrbye L, Onyeador IN, Phelan SM, van Ryn M. Contact and role modeling predict bias against lesbian and gay individuals among early-career physicians: a longitudinal study. Soc Sci Med. 2019;238:112422. https://doi.org/10.1016/j.socscimed.2019.112422.
78. Green TL, Vu H, Swan LET, Luo D, Hickman E, Plaisime M, Hagiwara N. Implicit and explicit racial prejudice among medical professionals: updated estimates from a population-based study. Lancet Reg Health Am. 2023;21:100489. https://doi.org/10.1016/j.lana.2023.100489.
79. Fernández CR, Silva D, Mancias P, Roldan EO, Sánchez JP. Hispanic identity and its inclusion in the race discrimination discourse in the United States. Acad Med. 2021;96(6):788–91. https://doi.org/10.1097/ACM.0000000000003904.
80. Nelson LR, Signorella ML, Botti KG. Accent, gender, and perceived competence. Hisp J Behav Sci. 2016;38:166–85.
81. Mpalirwa J, Lofters A, Nnorom O, Hanson MD. Patients, pride, and prejudice: exploring black ontarian physicians' experiences of racism and discrimination. Acad Med. 2020;95:S51–7. https://doi.org/10.1097/ACM.0000000000003648. (11S Association of American Medical Colleges Learn Serve Lead: Proceedings of the 59th Annual Research in Medical Education Presentations)
82. Filut A, Alvarez M, Carnes M. Discrimination toward physicians of color: a systematic review. J Natl Med Assoc. 2020;112(2):117–40. https://doi.org/10.1016/j.jnma.2020.02.008.
83. Isaac C, Lee B, Carnes M. Interventions that affect gender bias in hiring: a systematic review. Acad Med. 2009;84(10):1440–6. https://doi.org/10.1097/ACM.0b013e3181b6ba00.
84. Burke E, Heron EA, Hennessy M. Gender bias in academic medicine: a resumé study. BMC Med Educ. 2023;23(1):291. https://doi.org/10.1186/s12909-023-04192-6.
85. Hui K, Sukhera J, Vigod S, Taylor VH, Zaheer J. Recognizing and addressing implicit gender bias in medicine. CMAJ. 2020;192(42):E1269–70. https://doi.org/10.1503/cmaj.200286.
86. Gaiaschi C. Gender inequalities in medical careers: evidences from five hospitals in the Lombardy region. Ital J Gender-Specific Med. 2018;4:73–8.
87. Tricco AC, Bourgeault I, Moore A, Grunfeld E, Peer N, Straus SE. Advancing gender equity in medicine. CMAJ. 2021;193(7):E244–50. https://doi.org/10.1503/cmaj.200951.

88. Wijnen MN, Massen JJM, Kret ME. Gender bias in the allocation of student grants. Scientometrics. 2021;126:5477–88. https://doi.org/10.1007/s11192-021-03985-0.
89. Clayborne EP, Martin DR, Goett RR, Chandrasekaran EB, McGreevy J. Diversity pipelines: the rationale to recruit and support minority physicians. J Am Coll Emerg Phys Open. 2021;2(1):e12343. https://doi.org/10.1002/emp2.12343.
90. Laurencin CT, Murray M. An American crisis: the lack of black men in medicine. J Racial Ethn Health Disparities. 2017;4(3):317–21. https://doi.org/10.1007/s40615-017-0380-y.
91. Hall TR, Brown K. Diversity in radiology: the right thing to do, the smart thing to do. Pediatr Radiol. 2022;52(9):1711–8. https://doi.org/10.1007/s00247-022-05416-5.
92. Chapman CH, Hwang WT, Both S, Thomas CR Jr, Deville C. Current status of diversity by race, Hispanic ethnicity, and sex in diagnostic radiology. Radiology. 2014 Jan;270(1):232–40. https://doi.org/10.1148/radiol.13130101.
93. Seely JM. Women in radiology: challenges and opportunities. J Breast Imaging. 2024;6(5):539–46. https://doi.org/10.1093/jbi/wbae030.
94. Fichera G, Busch IM, Rimondini M, Motta R, Giraudo C. Is empowerment of female radiologists still needed? Findings of a systematic review. Int J Environ Res Public Health. 2021;18(4):1542. https://doi.org/10.3390/ijerph18041542.
95. Grimm LJ, Redmond RA, Campbell JC, Rosette AS. Gender and racial bias in radiology residency letters of recommendation. J Am Coll Radiol. 2020;17(1 Pt A):64–71. https://doi.org/10.1016/j.jacr.2019.08.008.
96. Tejani AS, Ng YS, Xi Y, Rayan JC. Understanding and mitigating bias in imaging artificial intelligence. Radiographics. 2024;44(5):e230067. https://doi.org/10.1148/rg.230067.
97. Ross AB, Kalia V, Chan BY, Li G. The influence of patient race on the use of diagnostic imaging in United States emergency departments: data from the National Hospital Ambulatory Medical Care survey. BMC Health Serv Res. 2020;20(1):840. https://doi.org/10.1186/s12913-020-05698-1.
98. Groen AM, Kraan R, Amirkhan SF, Daams JG, Maas M. A systematic review on the use of explainability in deep learning systems for computer aided diagnosis in radiology: limited use of explainable AI? Eur J Radiol. 2022;157:110592.
99. Sohn JH, Chen Y, Lituiev D, et al. Prediction of future healthcare expenses of patients from chest radiographs using deep learning: a pilot study. Sci Rep. 2022;12(1):8344.
100. Nikolic B. Racial Bias exacerbated through AI: an example using chest radiograph models. Radiology. 2023;309(2):e232666. https://doi.org/10.1148/radiol.232666.
101. Bachina P, Garin SP, Kulkarni P, Kanhere A, Sulam J, Parekh VS, Yi PH. Coarse race and ethnicity labels mask granular underdiagnosis disparities in deep learning models for chest radiograph diagnosis. Radiology. 2023;309(2):e231693. https://doi.org/10.1148/radiol.231693.
102. Curto G, Jojoa Acosta MF, Comim F, Garcia-Zapirain B. Are AI systems biased against the poor? A machine learning analysis using Word2Vec and GloVe embeddings. AI Soc. 2022:1–16. https://doi.org/10.1007/s00146-022-01494-z.
103. How Trump's DEI executive orders could impact healthcare. Emma Beavins Fierce Healthcare https://www.fiercehealthcare.com/regulatory/trumps-dei-executive-orders-could-impact-healthcare. Accessed on 9 Feb 2025.
104. "We are a target": scientific society under pressure after Trump DEI crackdown. Basilio Humberto. https://www.google.com/search?client=firefox-b-d&q=%E2%80%9CWe+are+a+target%E2%80%9D%3A+scientific+society+under+pressure+after+Trump+DEI+crackdown. Accessed on 9 Feb 2025.
105. Trump executive order puts STEM diversity efforts on hold. Virginia Gewin January 28, 2025. Science Insider. https://www.science.org/content/article/trump-executive-order-puts-stem-diversity-efforts-hold. Accessed on 9 Feb 2025.
106. Pratt-Chapman ML, Alpert AB, Castillo DA. Health outcomes of sexual and gender minorities after cancer: a systematic review. Syst Rev. 2021;10(1):183.
107. Cerdeña JP, Rehman T, Hardeman RR. Why bias matters in medicine: qualitative insights from anonymous, online reports. J Natl Med Assoc. 2020;112(1):6–14. https://doi.org/10.1016/j.jnma.2019.10.004.

Gender Competence in Clinical Medicine and Radiology 14

Bettina Pfleiderer

Gender competence in health care promotes equity in health outcomes [1].

14.1 Introduction

In recent years, the importance of the inclusion of gender competence in patient care has become increasingly recognized in clinical practice and medical education. Sex and gender aspects influence disease prevalence, symptom presentation, treatment response, patient–provider communication, health-seeking behavior, and access to care [2, 3]. Therefore, gender competence is a core competency, not an additional skill, for delivering equitable, evidence-based, and personalized medical care [1, 4].

Despite growing awareness, knowledge about gender aspect remains underrepresented in medicine and has not included sufficiently in many medical curricula. Still, traditional educational and clinical decision-making approaches often rely on male-centric research data and overlook the complex interplay between biological sex and sociocultural gender. This can result in diagnostic errors, suboptimal treatment, and reduced patient satisfaction, particularly among individuals whose health needs differ from the norm [2, 3].

14.1.1 Key Terms and Definitions

Gender competence is crucial to ensure that healthcare is medically appropriate and respectful of patients' diverse gender identities (Table 14.1). Gender roles, gendered stereotypes, and biases shape our daily clinical practice [5], how we are perceived

B. Pfleiderer (✉)
Research Group Cognition & Gender, Clinic of Radiology, Münster, Germany
e-mail: pfleide@uni-muenster.de

S. Keller-Yamamura, J. Yamamura (eds.), *Inclusive Radiology: Fostering Diversity and Equity in Academic and non-Academic Settings*,
https://doi.org/10.1007/978-3-032-05705-1_14

by others and how we interact with others (see Chap. 13). However, before diving into the topic of gender competence in medicine in more depth, it is important to present the key terms (Fig. 14.1).

14.1.1.1 Definitions

Table 14.1 presents the most important terms in the context of gender competence in healthcare. Gender intersects with other identities and shapes how we interact with patients [6].

Table 14.1 Definitions of terms of importance in gender competence

Term	Definition
Intersex	A general term for various conditions in which an individual is born with reproductive or sexual anatomy that doesn't fit typical definitions of male or female [9]
Gender identity	A person's deeply felt internal and individual experience of gender, which may or may not correspond with the sex assigned at birth [10]
Cisgender	A person whose gender identity aligns with the sex they were assigned at birth [11]
Transgender	A person whose gender identity differs from the sex they were assigned at birth. This includes those who transition and those who do not [11]
Gender-fluid	Individuals with a gender identity or expression that may shift over time or in different contexts, moving between genders or outside traditional categories [12]
Agender	A person who identifies as having no gender or being without gender identity [13]
Genderqueer	An umbrella term for identities that are not exclusively male or female; may combine, reject, or transcend binary gender categories [12]
Gender-neutral	Describes language, spaces, or roles that avoid distinguishing by sex or gender, aiming for inclusivity across gender identities [14]
Gender role	Societal norms and expectations about behaviors, responsibilities, and activities deemed appropriate based on perceived gender [15]

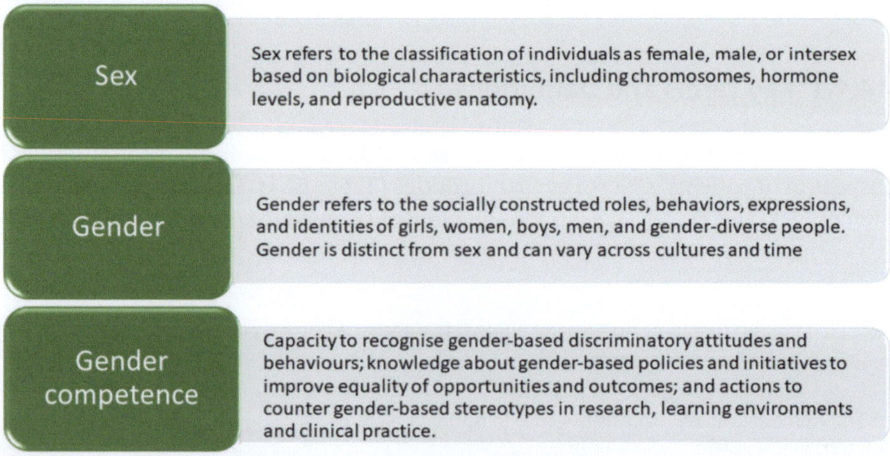

Fig. 14.1 Key terms of gender competence in medicine [1–4, 6]

14.1.1.2 Intersectionality in Clinical Care

> Intersectionality in clinical care can be defined as a framework that recognizes and addresses the manner in which an individual's multiple identities (e.g., race, gender, class, age, sexual orientation, ability, religion, immigration status) intersect to create unique experiences of privilege and discrimination, which ultimately impact an individual's access to healthcare and health outcomes [6–8].

Intersectionality addresses the unique and overlapping experiences of individuals who belong to multiple marginalized groups [7, 8]. To illustrate this point, patients from marginalized communities may encounter a greater number of healthcare barriers when compared to those from non-marginalized communities (LGBTQIA+ (Lesbians, Gay people, Bisexual people, Transsexual/Transgender people, Queer people, Intersex people, and Asexual people) or migrants). LGBTQIA+ females of color face more challenges as white LGBTQIA+ females.

14.2 Gender Competence in Medical Care

In the context of clinical medicine and individualized patient care, **gender competence** refers to the ability of healthcare professionals to recognize, respect, and address the gender-related needs, identities, and experiences of patients. Gender influences risks, treatment responses, and health behaviors [3]. For example, symptoms can differ between men and women, as well as women are more likely to experience adverse drug reactions than men, a difference that has been partly attributed to the fact that clinical drug trials have historically been conducted predominantly in healthy young males, often excluding women due to hormonal variability or reproductive concerns [16]. As a result, sex-based pharmacokinetic and pharmacodynamic differences have often been overlooked, leading to inappropriate dosing or underestimated risks for women across many drug classes [16]. Gender-competent care aims to recognize and dismantle these systemic inequities [3, 17].

Historically, healthcare systems have operated within a binary model of gender, failing to reflect the diverse gender identities of patients [18]. Gender competence includes understanding identities such as nonbinary, transgender, genderqueer, and gender-fluid [12], and using inclusive communication [10]. Transgender individuals, for instance, may require hormone therapy or gender-affirming procedures, which will affect treatment, risk for certain diseases and care in general [19].

14.2.1 Why Does Gender Competence Matter?

Gender-competent care relates to care that is both ethically sound and legally compliant, with the objective of ensuring nondiscrimination in healthcare [20]. The provision of gender-competent care has been demonstrated to enhance adherence and satisfaction, thereby improving overall health outcomes [2, 3], as well as to reduction of health disparities. Gender-competent professionals in the medical sector are able to ensure that all aspects of a patient's sex and gender identity are considered when making medical decisions, leading to superior health outcomes. Furthermore, patients who feel understood are more likely to seek care and participate in their treatment plans, especially those from marginalized groups [10]. This is particularly significant for improving the health of LGBTQIA+ individuals, who frequently encounter obstacles in accessing adequate healthcare services [19]. Healthcare professionals have an ethical and legal obligation to provide care that is free from discrimination.

14.3 Gender Competence in the Context of Radiology

Despite the perception of radiology as a neutral, image-based specialty, the influence of sex and gender aspects on imaging choices, interpretation of imaging results, should be considered. The influence of sex on anatomy, pathology, and clinical presentation can have a significant impact on image interpretation, protocol selection, and patient communication [3].

14.3.1 Female and Male Kidneys Differ

There is ample documentation of marked differences in kidney size between males and females, with implications for the pharmacokinetics of substances eliminated via the kidneys, including iodinated and gadolinium-based contrast agents.

14.3.1.1 Structural Sex Differences

When adjusted for body surface area (BSA) or height, male kidneys tend to be larger than female kidneys in terms of size and relative volume. A study of autopsy samples from Switzerland revealed that the mean mass of male kidneys was approximately 25% greater than that of female kidneys, with this difference being statistically significant even after adjustment for body surface area [21, 22]. The number of nephrons (functional units of the kidney) and glomerular size also differ. It has been demonstrated that women generally possess a lower number of nephrons or smaller glomeruli in comparison to men, which has been hypothesized to result in a reduction of total filtration capacity [23].

14.3.1.2 Renal Function and Clearance Differences

These anatomical differences result in important functional differences. Women typically exhibit lower absolute glomerular filtration rate (GFR) and reduced renal plasma flow, combined with higher renovascular resistance [22, 24]. These differences are not solely due to body size but may also be influenced by hormonal factors such as estrogen levels, which modulate vascular tone and renal hemodynamic [25].

Table 14.2 Structural and functional differences between female and male kidneys

Feature	Male vs female	Impact on agent clearance
Kidney volume/weight [21, 22]	~25% larger in males (absolute & relative)	Larger renal capacity → faster clearance in men
Nephron number/ glomerular volume [23]	Higher in males (fewer, smaller in females)	Higher filtration → faster clearance in men
GFR and renal plasma flow [22, 24]	Higher in males	Higher filtration → faster clearance in men
Hormonal/drug effects [25, 26]	Estrogen/ NSAIDs lower clearance	May lead to reduced elimination in women

NSAID nonsteroidal anti-inflammatory drug, *GFR* glomerular filtration rate

14.3.1.3 Contrast Agent Pharmacokinetics

Contrast agents used in imaging (e.g., computer tomography or MRI) are primarily eliminated via renal excretion, and the efficiency of this process is heavily dependent on kidney function and blood flow. Studies suggest that drugs and agents cleared renally tend to have a slower clearance rate in women due to lower GFR and renal blood flow [26]. Additionally, common medications and hormonal therapies—such as oral contraceptives or estrogen replacement therapy—can further reduce GFR, exacerbating the slower elimination in females [26].

To summarize (Table 14.2), in female patients, particularly those with compromised renal function or on concurrent medications, contrast agents may persist longer in the bloodstream. The impact may be low in healthy individuals; however, in women who have additional factors, such as hormonal therapy or on nonsteroidal anti-inflammatory drugs, this may result in a longer retention time, which could potentially influence the timing of imaging or increase the risk of contrast-induced nephropathy. It is incumbent upon radiologists to be aware of these aspects and to adjust imaging protocols accordingly.

14.4 Practical Steps to Achieve Gender Competence in Clinical Care and Radiology

14.4.1 Curriculum Design and Faculty Training

Healthcare professionals should receive ongoing education about gender identity, expression, and related health issues [10]. This training should include the influence of gender on physical and mental well-being, and the necessity of inclusive communication. It is imperative that particular emphasis is placed on respectful communication. This encompasses the respectful exploration of gender identity and the utilization of appropriate pronouns, while avoiding assumptions [10]. Awareness of cultural and social dimensions of gender enhances patient engagement and trust.

This can be achieved by integrating gender competence into radiology training curricula, including:

- Draft of case studies with diverse gender presentations with a view to showcasing a range of gender presentations:
  - A positive example of gender-competent radiological experience.
  - A missed diagnosis due to wrong assumptions about sex/gender.
  - An imaging challenge due to altered anatomy.
  - A case involving transgender persons with clinical information, including the impact of gender-affirming hormones and how to tailor imaging protocols to transgender patients.
- Modules on respectful communication with transgender patients.
- Teaching of radiological relevant sex-based anatomy and the impact of pathological variations on radiological examinations. Radiological procedures frequently rely on sex-assigned protocols, which may not accurately reflect a patient's current anatomy or healthcare requirements. For instance, a transgender woman may still require prostate imaging, whereas a transgender man may require breast or pelvic imaging, depending on their surgical and hormonal status.

Educate radiologists on the potential implications of hormone therapy in transgender patients, thereby preventing misinterpretation of imaging results. The impact of gender-affirming hormone therapy on tissue density, organ appearance, and risk profiles is a multifaceted area of research. It has been demonstrated that estrogen therapy may result in an increased risk of developing thromboembolic disease, as evidenced by the presence of visible lesions on computer tomography or Doppler ultrasound scans. In contrast, testosterone therapy has been observed to exert an impact on muscle and bone tissue [27]. Procedures such as mammography, pelvic ultrasound, or scrotal ultrasound have been found to cause distress for transgender and nonbinary patients. Gender-competent radiology encompasses respectful communication, consent practices, and the provision of gender-congruent chaperones or staff when feasible [8].

14.4.2 Creating Safe and Inclusive Environments

Healthcare facilities should implement policies that create a welcoming environment for all patients, irrespective of gender. This could involve displaying nondiscriminatory signage, providing gender-neutral restrooms, and offering staff training to promote respectful and inclusive interactions with all patients. This can be achieved by

- Respectful use of pronouns.
- Gaining informed consent with sensitivity to gender identity.
- Offering same-gender technicians when preferred.

14.4.3 Gender-Inclusive Radiological Data Collection

Healthcare systems should collect and record gender identity data in a manner that respects the individual and allows for a comprehensive understanding of patient demographics It is imperative that this information is utilized to enhance patient care and ensure that all gender identities are adequately represented in healthcare [28]. Radiology departments and practices should therefore advocate for inclusive documentation in PACS and RIS systems and to support gender-diverse representation as a variable in imaging research and AI datasets [17, 18]. It is generally considered good practice for the documentation of surgical history and gender identity to be included in radiological referrals. In cases involving transgender patients, radiologists are advised to remind referring physicians of the importance of this aspect of the referral process.

14.4.4 Collaborating with Experts

It is of importance that radiological staff collaborate with specialists in transgender healthcare, and other gender-related services as required. The establishment of networks with these experts has the potential to enhance the quality of care for patients with complex gender-related radiological needs.

14.5 Conclusions

The ability to demonstrate gender competence in the clinical medicine setting is of paramount importance when providing individualized patient care. By understanding and respecting the diversity of gender identities, as well as addressing the unique healthcare needs that arise from gender-related factors. It is evident that gender competence is in line with a patient-centered care model, which prioritizes individualized health requirements as opposed to group stereotypes. As radiology becomes increasingly central to diagnosis and treatment, there is a need for gender-informed imaging protocols and inclusive communication to become standard practice. The adoption of gender-competent practices by healthcare professionals will be fostering greater trust between patients and practitioners. This, in turn, has been shown to reduce disparities in health outcomes.

References

1. Fisher J. Gender competence and mental health promotion. World Psychiatry. 2020;19(1):34–5. https://doi.org/10.1002/wps.20694.
2. Becher E, Oertelt-Prigione S. The impact of sex and gender in medicine and pharmacology. Handb Exp Pharmacol. 2023;282:3–23. https://doi.org/10.1007/164_2023_68.
3. Mauvais-Jarvis F, Bairey Merz N, Barnes PJ, Brinton RD, Carrero J-J, DeMeo DL, et al. Sex and gender: modifiers of health, disease, and medicine. Lancet. 2020;396(10250):565–82. https://doi.org/10.1016/S0140-6736(20)31561-0.
4. Mahr F, Dalke K, Roden RC, Keisling AK, Petrovic-Dovat L. Gender competence in medical education. Clin Teach. 2021;18:490–3. https://doi.org/10.1016/S0140-6736(20)31561-0.
5. Cunningham GB, Wicker P. Sexual harassment and implicit gender-career biases negatively impact women's life expectancy in the US: a state-level analysis, 2011–2019. BMC Public Health. 2024;24(1):1115. https://doi.org/10.1186/s12889-024-18450-9.

6. Wilson Y, White A, Jefferson A, Danis M. Intersectionality in clinical medicine: the need for a conceptual framework. AJOB. 2019;19(2):8–19. https://doi.org/10.1080/15265161.2018.1557275.
7. Subramaniapillai S, Galea LAM, Einstein G, de Lange A-MG. Sex and gender in health research: intersectionality matters. Front Neuroendocrinol. 2024;72:101104. https://doi.org/10.1016/j.yfrne.2023.101104.
8. Barned C, Lajoie C, Racine E. Addressing the practical implications of intersectionality in clinical medicine: ethical, embodied and institutional dimensions. AJOB. 2019;19(2):27–9. https://doi.org/10.1080/15265161.2018.1557278.
9. Hughes IA, Houk C, Fau-Ahmed SF, Ahmed Sf Fau-Lee PA, Lee PA. Consensus statement on management of intersex disorders. Arch Dis Child. 2006;91:554–63. https://doi.org/10.1136/adc.2006.098319.
10. American Psychological A. Guidelines for psychological practice with transgender and gender nonconforming people. Am Psychol. 2015;70:832–64. https://doi.org/10.1037/a0039906.
11. Darwin H. Challenging the cisgender/transgender binary: nonbinary people and the transgender label. G & S. 2020;34(3):357–80. https://doi.org/10.1177/0891243220912256.
12. Richards C, Bouman WP, Seal L, Barker M-J, Nieder TO, T'Sjoen G. Non-binary or genderqueer genders. Int Rev Psychiatr. 2016;28(1):95–102. https://doi.org/10.3109/09540261.2015.1106446.
13. Morrison T, Dinno A, Salmon T. The erasure of intersex, transgender, nonbinary, and agender experiences through misuse of sex and gender in health research. Am J Epidemiol. 2021;190(12):2712–7. https://doi.org/10.1093/aje/kwab221.
14. Sarrasin O, Gabriel U, Gygax P. Sexism and attitudes toward gender-neutral language. Swiss J Psychol. 2012;71(3):113–24. https://doi.org/10.1024/1421-0185/a000078.
15. Eagly AH. Sex differences in social behavior: a social-role interpretation. 1st ed. Hillsdale: Psychology Press; 1987. https://doi.org/10.4324/9780203781906.
16. Zucker I, Prendergast BJ. Sex differences in pharmacokinetics predict adverse drug reactions in women. Biol Sex Differ. 2020;11(12):32. https://doi.org/10.1186/s13293-020-00308-5.
17. Springer KW, Hankivsky O, Benoit C. Policy and research priorities for advancing gender equity in medicine. Soc Sci Med. 2012;74(11):1817–24. https://doi.org/10.1016/j.socscimed.2011.11.009.
18. Springer KW, Hankivsky O, Bates LM. Gender and health: relational, intersectional, and biosocial approaches. Soc Sci Med. 2012;74(11):1661–6. https://doi.org/10.1016/j.socscimed.2011.08.009.
19. Winter S, Diamond M, Green J, Karasic D, Reed T, Whittle S, et al. Transgender people: health at the margins of society. Lancet. 2016;388(10042):390–400. https://doi.org/10.1016/S0140-6736(16)00683-8.
20. MacNaughton G. Untangling equality and non-discrimination to promote the right to health for all. HHR. 2009;11(2):47–63. http://www.jstor.org/stable/25653102. Accessed 1 Aug. 2025
21. Kalucki SA, Lardi C, Garessus J, Kfoury A, Grabherr S, Burnier M, et al. Reference values and sex differences in absolute and relative kidney size. A Swiss autopsy study BMC Nephrol. 2020;21(1):289. https://doi.org/10.1186/s12882-020-01946-y.
22. Dabers T, Sass P, Fechner F, Weyer J, Völzke H, Mahnken AH, et al. Age- and sex-specific reference values for renal volume and association with risk factors for chronic kidney disease in a general population—an MRI-based study. J Clin Med. 2024;13(3):769. https://doi.org/10.3390/jcm13030769.
23. Nyengaard J, Bendtsen T. Number and size of glomeruli in human kidneys: influence of age, sex, and body size. Anat Rec. 1993;235(2):255–62. https://doi.org/10.1002/ar.1092350210.
24. Neugarten J, Golestaneh L. Gender and the prevalence and progression of renal disease. AKDH. 2013;20(5):390–5. https://doi.org/10.1053/j.ackd.2013.05.005.
25. Silbiger S, Neugarten J. Gender and human chronic renal disease. Gend Med. 2008;5(Suppl A):S3–S10. https://doi.org/10.1016/j.genm.2008.03.002.
26. Soldin OP, Mattison DR. Sex differences in pharmacokinetics and pharmacodynamics. Clin Pharmacokinet. 2009;48(3):143–57. https://doi.org/10.2165/00003088-200948030-00001.

27. Griggs RC, Kingston W, Jozefowicz RF, Herr BE, Forbes G, Halliday D. Effect of testosterone on muscle mass and muscle protein synthesis. J Appl Physiol. 1985;66:498–503. https://doi.org/10.1152/jappl.1989.66.1.498.
28. Day S, Mason R, Tannenbaum C, Rochon PA. Essential metrics for assessing sex & gender integration in health research proposals involving human participants. PLoS One. 2017;12(8):e0182812. https://doi.org/10.1371/journal.pone.0182812.

How to Increase Diversity and Inclusion in the Radiological Department 15

Isolde Martina Busch, Michela Rimondini, and Chiara Giraudo

> We all should know that diversity makes for a rich tapestry, and we must understand that all the threads of the tapestry are equal in value no matter what their color. (Maya Angelou)

15.1 Introduction

Diversity, equity, and inclusion (DEI) refers to "*the idea that all people should have equal rights and treatment and be welcomed and included, so that they do not experience any disadvantage because of belonging to a particular group, and that each person should be given the same opportunities as others according to their needs*" [1].

DEI initiatives have been shown to have a positive impact not only on individuals but on organizations and communities as a whole, with positive outcomes like an improved competitive position, agility, and innovation [2, 3]. In healthcare, this impact is especially important [4]. A diverse workforce contributes to improved health equity, social justice, and financial health [5–7]. It allows for more inclusive patient care, where various perspectives lead to better outcomes and more culturally competent services [8]. Additionally, it supports the expansion of access to healthcare careers for women and underrepresented minorities in medicine (URiM) [5–7]. URiM is defined by the Association of American Medical Colleges (AAMC) as

I. M. Busch · M. Rimondini
Department of Neurosciences, Section of Clinical Psychology, Biomedicine, and Movement Sciences, University of Verona, Verona, Italy
e-mail: isoldemartina.busch@univr.it; michela.rimondini@univr.it

C. Giraudo (✉)
Department of Cardiac, Thoracic, Vascular Sciences and Public Health—DCTV, Unit of Advanced Clinical and Translational Imaging, University of Padova, Padova, Italy
e-mail: chiara.giraudo@unipd.it

S. Keller-Yamamura, J. Yamamura (eds.), *Inclusive Radiology: Fostering Diversity and Equity in Academic and non-Academic Settings*,
https://doi.org/10.1007/978-3-032-05705-1_15

"those racial and ethnic populations that are underrepresented in the medical profession relative to their numbers in the general population" [9]. However, several institutions and scholars have advocated for expanding the definition of URiM beyond race and ethnicity to include factors such as socioeconomic status, LGBTQIA+ identity, and disabilities [10, 11]. In this chapter, we adopt this broader definition of URiM, incorporating these additional communities.

Radiology is one of the medical fields that sees only a slow advancement in increasing representation for women and underrepresented minorities [5]. Fostering DEI in radiology, as in other fields, is essential for improving workforce representation and ensuring that it remains a dynamic specialty capable of meeting the challenges of a diverse patient population [12].

However, recently, there has been a widespread effort to roll back DEI measures on a massive scale, with major corporations like Amazon and Meta preemptively complying with the shifting political landscape [13–15]. For instance, over 8000 pages related to diversity, gender, and the climate crisis were removed from public websites, potentially limiting access to critical health and environmental information [16, 17]. However, this action was recently challenged in court, resulting in a ruling that key public health agencies must restore previously removed websites and datasets that had been taken down without notice [18]. These ongoing legal and political battles highlight that DEI measures are not assured and when challenged, they can have far-reaching consequences for healthcare and scientific institutions.

With radiology playing a vital role in patient care and medical research, upholding and expanding DEI principles across all levels is key to fostering a more inclusive and equitable environment for both healthcare providers and patients. In the following sections, we highlight key areas where DEI initiatives have already been successfully implemented or should be integrated within radiological settings. These include departmental policies that promote equity and inclusivity, educational and training programs, mentorship opportunities, workplace culture, clinical practice, health equity measures, community engagement, the work of radiology societies and organizations, and research.

15.2 Advancing DEI in the Radiological Department

To effectively advance DEI in the radiology department, it is essential to first gain a comprehensive understanding of the current state of DEI initiatives, challenges, and opportunities. Assessing the existing landscape allows for the identification of gaps, the evaluation of ongoing efforts, and the development of targeted strategies to foster a more inclusive and equitable environment. Useful tools to examine these aspects can be surveys of both staff and patients as well as the implementation of audits. For instance, Perchik et al. [19] describe the successful performance of an LGBTQ inclusion audit to review existing department policies regarding LGBTQ issues.

Forming a dedicated DEI committee within the radiology department can provide structured oversight for such surveys and audits and drive the respective implementation of measures to address the gaps [5, 20]. Narayan and colleagues [20] from the Mass General's Department of Radiology first performed a gap analysis and an assessment of the strengths and weaknesses of their center, which then served as a guidance for the implementation of a radiology departmental DEI committee, comprised of a steering committee and four task forces focusing on education, research, patient experience, and workforce development. The authors underline that strong leadership support and broad staff engagement are crucial for establishing a successful DEI committee and that aligning its initiatives with departmental and institutional goals ensures its growth and effectiveness [20].

Assessing the DEI situation in the radiology department just once is not sufficient. Progress should be continuously monitored, under the supervision of the DEI committee, and policies and interventions should be refined over time.

15.2.1 Departmental Policies and Programs

Important areas benefitting from DEI policies include family-supportive strategies, flexible work opportunities, and programs ensuring fair distribution of promotions [21, 22].

Family leave programs, including paid parental leave and childcare support, as well as paid medical leave not only promote a good work–life balance but can also improve health outcomes for the entire family [23, 24]. Additionally, healthcare institutions benefit since such policies help in attracting and retaining talent, fostering a positive workplace culture, boosting employee morale and productivity, and reducing overall costs [24].

Moreover, flexible work arrangements can promote better work–life integration, reduce job-related stress, and enhance job satisfaction and emotional well-being [25]. Remote work options in radiology departments, particularly within academic institutions, have become increasingly prevalent, such as at University Hospital Essen in Germany [26].

To promote fair career advancement, it is essential to implement transparent promotion programs with clearly defined criteria, together with mentorship and sponsorship initiatives [27]. Widespread implementation of these programs is crucial, especially considering the ongoing challenges faced by minorities. For instance, research has shown that anti-Black racism continues to contribute to career disadvantages and the underrepresentation of Black physicians [28].

15.3 Training and Education

15.3.1 Mentorship Programs

Given the increasing challenges in healthcare, mentorship can be seen as a crucial element for career success, personal development, and well-being of academic radiologists [29, 30]. It not only aids in career development and job satisfaction but might also play a role in preventing burnout [19, 31]. Creating a diverse network of mentors—across different levels and backgrounds—can better support faculty, especially women and URiM. These groups, who often lack mentorship opportunities, stand to benefit most from having access to mentors who can emphatically address their specific challenges and needs [29, 30, 32]. Mentors who belong themselves to minorities or marginalized groups can lead by example and enhance mentee's confidence, self-esteem, and sense of belonging [32]. Radiology departments should therefore establish mentoring programs that emphasize diversity and ensure that all faculty members have equal opportunities for professional and personal growth.

Several mentorship programs for women and minority radiology faculty have been already successfully implemented, such as the National Virtual Mentorship Program for women, international medical graduate students and individuals from URiM [33], the Mentorship and Networking group for women in radiology [34], and the Leadership Intervention to Further the Training of Female Faculty (LIFT-OFF) in Radiology [35]. A study on the LGBTQ+ mentorship program at the Schulich School of Medicine & Dentistry, Western University (Ontario, Canada) [36], found that LGBTQ+ mentees reported increased optimism about their careers and a stronger sense of community. The program also had a positive impact on mentors, helping them view themselves as role models and fostering a greater sense of belonging within the faculty [36].

15.3.2 Training Programs

Tailored training for radiological staff should comprehensively address key topics such as diversity, equity, and inclusion, fostering respect and collaboration within the department, and tackling the unique challenges faced by female and URiM colleagues [21, 37]. Training could include interactive sessions on recognizing and mitigating biases both toward colleagues and patients, understanding the impact of microaggressions, and developing strategies to build allyship and create a more supportive work environment. Role-plays, scenarios, and case studies can be particularly effective tools for engaging staff, encouraging introspection and reflection, and increasing empathy [38–41]. For instance, the Department of Radiology at the University of Wisconsin–Madison provides DEI-focused training sessions, such as workshops on combating microaggressions in the workplace and bootcamps aimed at fostering inclusive practices within radiology [42].

In addition, specialized workshops should address the issue of workplace violence, including patient-to-worker and worker-to-worker incidents [43], with particular attention to how racism, sexism, and hostility toward LGBTQIA+ individuals might fuel such violence.

These workshops could focus on conflict resolution techniques, violence prevention, and other precautionary measures applying scenario-based training role-playing exercises, and group case discussions [43–45].

To ensure lasting impact, these topics should also be embedded into medical school curricula and residency programs, as already done by several medical schools and radiological departments [42, 46, 47]. For instance, the Diversity, Equity, Inclusion, Access and Social Justice Curriculum at the University of Michigan Medical School has demonstrated success by incorporating DEI-focused education into early medical training, equipping future radiologists with the skills to navigate and address these challenges in their interactions with colleagues and diverse patient population from the very start of their careers [46].

Such initiatives aim not only to create a more inclusive and respectful workplace culture but also to improve access to care for female patients and individuals from minority and marginalized groups, enhancing the quality of care they receive.

15.4 Psychological Support Resources

We also advocate for substantial investments in emotional and mental health resources within radiology departments. These efforts aim not only to address the high rates of burnout among radiologists but also to offer a safe and supportive environment for female and URiM radiology faculty and trainees who may face implicit biases and prejudice, feelings of isolation at the workplace, and, at times, discriminatory interactions with patients, which may lead to emotional distress [12, 19, 32, 48–50]. To address these challenges, it is essential to offer counseling services, access to short-term psychotherapy, or referrals to other mental health centers when needed, as well as preventive psychological interventions aimed at fostering resilience and a sense of belonging.

Psychological support is very important also to support victims of workplace violence—whether from patients or colleagues—since such episodes can have a significant impact on radiological staff [43], particularly on female and minority staff, who may already face systemic challenges in the workplace. In this case, it is particularly important to emphasize the confidentiality of available support services to encourage victims to come forward, as being a victim of workplace violence carries significant stigma [43, 51]. Existing psychological programs should be expanded and tailored to address all various needs [43, 51], considering the intersection of workplace violence, gender, and minority status.

To provide holistic and compassionate care, it is crucial that easily accessible, confidential psychological support services are also available for patients and their caregivers who may feel discriminated or treated unfairly by radiological staff due to their gender identity, sexual orientation, race, or ethnicity.

15.5 Clinical Practice

Health disparities in radiology, often driven by structural barriers related to a patient's socioeconomic background, location, or demographic traits, can arise at any stage of the healthcare continuum—from screenings and monitoring to follow-up care [52, 53]. Lawson et al. emphasize that disparities in access and utilization of care at earlier stages can lead to compounding inequities over time [53]. Improving access to imaging that directly impact patient outcomes, such as timely breast screenings, is therefore crucial [53]. One approach to addressing these disparities is strengthening collaborations between different healthcare facilities, such as academic medical centers and rural hospitals to expand access to specialized care [54].

While these disparities affect many populations, certain groups face unique barriers to radiological care. In particular, transgender and nonbinary patients often experience stigmatization and discrimination within healthcare settings [55, 56]. A study by Grimstad et al. of a sample of 363 transgender and nonbinary individuals showed that approximately 70.8% had encountered negative experiences during imaging procedures [55]. To address these issues, it is essential for radiological departments to create welcoming environments, practice cultural humility, and stay informed about current guidelines related to this patient group [56].

15.6 Advancing DEI in Societies and Academia beyond the Radiological Department

It is not only important to diversify the radiological workplace itself, but also to promote diversity, equity, and inclusion in radiological societies and across the academic landscape of radiology.

15.6.1 Radiological Societies and Organizations

While some radiological societies still need to invest more in this area, many have made significant progress in advancing DEI in radiology. In recent years, dedicated committees have been established to raise awareness about DEI, diversify the radiological workforce and leadership, and advance health equity along with value-based healthcare. Examples include the *Committee on Diversity, Equity, and Inclusion* (CDEI) [57] and the *Health Equity Committee* (HEC) of the *Radiological Society of North America* (RSNA) [58], the *Diversity, Equity & Inclusion Committee* of the International Skeletal Society (ISS) [59], the *Equity, Diversity, and Inclusion Subcommittee* of the European Society of Radiology (ESR) [60], the *Equality, Diversity and Inclusion Taskforce* of the Royal College of Radiologists (RCR) [61], and the *Committee on Diversity, Equity and Inclusion* of the Society of Abdominal Radiology (SAR) [62]. Moreover, various societies are actively promoting DEI activities such as congress sessions and exhibits, symposia, online learning courses, and webinars. For instance, the European Society of Breast Imaging (EUSOBI) has announced a 2025 webinar highlighting recent advancements in breast imaging for male and transgender patients [63]. Similarly, the International Society for Magnetic Resonance in Medicine (ISMRM) and the RSNA offer a range of DEI resources on their website [57, 58, 64].

The integration of DEI principles and the commitment to delivering equitable patient care for everyone have even been recognized as one of the five essential goals in RSNA's Strategic Plan, set to direct the organization from 2024 through 2029 [65]. In addition to the initiatives mentioned above, the RSNA organizes events aimed at introducing high school students and recent college graduates to career opportunities in radiology. Furthermore, the RSNA's R&E Foundation offers research grants specifically for medical students from minority backgrounds [57].

Several radiological societies have conducted surveys to assess DEI issues among their members [66–69]. For instance, a study by Bredella & Chung [67] regarding the perception of equity and respect in the workplace and within the Society of Skeletal Radiology (SSR) found that participants considered women and individuals from minority groups as underrepresented in the SSR and facing greater obstacles and receiving less respect in their work environments than their male, nonminority counterparts. Further, a recent survey addressed to members of the ESSR by Giraudo et al. [66], highlights the ongoing underrepresentation of women and the need to improve gender equity within the organization. However, the survey also revealed encouraging signs of a tangible reduction in the gender gap.

Further, to advance healthcare equity in diagnostic imaging, leading organizations and societies—such as the American College of Radiology, the Radiological Society of North America, the Society of Nuclear Medicine and Molecular Imaging, and the American Society of Radiologic Technologists—have come together to form the Radiology Health Equity Coalition. This initiative focuses on gathering and sharing material, supporting underserved communities, and enhance access to imaging services [70].

15.6.2 Conferences

To improve diversity at radiological conferences, several strategies can be employed. For instance, increasing the number of women on selection panels has proven effective in increasing female representation among speakers, as a study on scientific medical conferences by Salem et al. [71] highlighted. Efforts should also focus on fostering environments that encourage female participation. For instance, women in chair positions or opening questions from women significantly increase women's engagement in Q&A sessions [71]. Advocacy by male allies, as emphasized in the UN's "HeForShe" campaign, is also crucial in fostering inclusivity [72, 73]. Comparable strategies can undoubtedly be used to enhance inclusivity for the LGBTQIA+ community, racial and ethnic groups, and people with disabilities [74].

As noted by Prathivadi Bhayankaram & Prathivadi Bhayankaram [74], both speakers and delegates have an important role in promoting diversity. For instance, invited speakers and delegates can ask about the diversity of panels and emphasize its significance and can encourage organizers to prioritize diverse representation [74]. The authors also emphasize that scientific journals can play an important role in raising awareness and promoting diversity, citing *The Lancet* as an example. The journal has committed to a diversity pledge, vowing to no longer participate in so-called "manels"—panels composed entirely of men. This sets a standard that other journals could follow as well [74, 75].

Clearly, also offering symposia, workshops, and other events specifically focused on DEI, as already proposed by radiological societies mentioned above, helps to create more equitable and inclusive spaces for all participants.

Furthermore, conference organizers should more frequently invite patients, especially those from underserved populations and minority groups, as speakers or panel members and consider opening the congress to them as participants. This would improve patient empowerment and reflect the medical community's commitment to improve access to healthcare spaces and foster inclusivity. While specific instances of patients serving as keynote speakers at imaging conferences are not widely documented, a notable example is the 2024 Molecular Imaging Symposium: Dennis Organ, a patient advocate and co-leader of the Pacific Northwest Carcinoid NET Support Group, delivered a keynote speech in which he shared his experience with imaging and theranostics services [76].

15.6.3 Research

Diverse research teams in healthcare and radiology are essential for fostering innovation, improving patient outcomes, and ensuring equitable representation in the field [54, 77–80]. A diverse group of researchers brings varied perspectives, leading to more comprehensive and inclusive research. Moreover, actively involving patients in research, particularly those from underserved populations, helps address diverse healthcare needs, enhances the relevance of findings, and promotes patient empowerment [52, 54, 80–82]. Patient empowerment, a crucial aspect of patient-centered healthcare, fosters autonomy and can also lead to improved health outcomes, such as increased patient compliance [82–84]. An effective approach to engage marginalized population is community-based participatory research. This method involves the collaboration with community members throughout the entire research process, ensuring that studies are culturally sensitive and relevant to the community's needs [80].

By incorporating previously excluded voices—both within the radiological workforce and among patients—research can expand to include topics such as DEI and health equity, ultimately contributing to more equitable healthcare outcomes.

Equitably offering grant support to female and URiM researchers is also crucial for driving meaningful change. For example, a systematic review by Fichera et al. [21] found that men reported receiving grant support more often and secured a higher number of grants than women. However, specific data comparing grant success rates between LGBTQIA+ researchers and their cisgender, heterosexual counterparts in radiology are currently lacking. Similarly, comprehensive statistics on grant funding disparities between racial or ethnic minority researchers and white researchers in radiology are limited. Regarding medical sciences more in general, a recent report from 2023 from the National Institutes of Health (NIH) indicated that, despite slight improvements in overall funding and success rates, a persistent funding gap remains between Black and white applicants [85].

The abovementioned systematic review also revealed that women were underrepresented on the editorial boards of radiology journals [21, 86–88]. Additionally, among four high-ranking radiology journals—*Radiology, American Journal of Roentgenology, JACR,* and *Academic Radiology*—no woman had ever served as chief editor [21, 88]. However, there is a notable lack of specific studies examining the representation of LGBTQIA+ individuals as well as the racial composition of editorial boards in radiology journals, highlighting the need for more comprehensive studies in this area to understand and address potential disparities in these influential positions. Although a study by White et al. [89] focused on surgical journals, it underscores the broader issue of underrepresentation of racial minorities in medical editorial leadership. The authors assessed diversity among editorial boards in surgical research found that only 2.9% of board members were Black and 3.3% were Hispanic, despite these groups comprising larger proportions of the general population.

When communicating research findings, researchers should be aware that language shapes our perception and thus follow established guidelines for unbiased and nonhandicapping language, such as the *bias-free language guidelines* in the seventh edition of the Publication Manual of the American Psychological Association (APA) [90] and the *Inclusive Language Guide* by the APA [91]. For instance, the Inclusive Language Guide explains why certain terms can be harmful and offers more inclusive alternatives. It is not exhaustive but serves to increase awareness and promote culturally sensitive terminology and encourages the use of specific, respectful terms that align with how individuals self-identify, while remaining open to learning and adapting [91].

Moreover, to make radiological research accessible to individuals with varying levels of health literacy, it is important to use plain-language resources [92]. This approach empowers patients, their families, caregivers, and the general public, while also strengthening shared decision-making [92].

15.7 Final Considerations

In conclusion, fostering diversity and inclusion in radiology—and beyond—requires a multifaceted approach that addresses individual, institutional, and societal levels [32]. Prejudice and discrimination against women and other marginalized groups are deeply ingrained in society, and systemic barriers persist within radiology, affecting both patients and underrepresented professionals, including women and URiM radiologists.

We call on the radiological community to stand firm against global pushback on DEI initiatives, recognizing the profound implications for public health, scientific progress, and democratic discourse. Rather than retreating, we advocate for expanding the promising approaches outlined earlier, including inclusive hiring practices, equitable departmental policies, substantial investment in mental health resources, ongoing education on bias and cultural competency, and improved healthcare access for marginalized patient groups.

By prioritizing these efforts, radiology departments and the broader radiological community can promote personal growth and professional well-being among their workforce, enhance team performance, drive innovation, improve patient care, and ensure the field truly reflects the diverse communities it serves.

References

1. Cambridge Dictionary. Diversity, equity and inclusion [cited 2025 Feb 13]. Available from: https://dictionary.cambridge.org/dictionary/english/diversity-equity-and-inclusion
2. Milanesi C. The business impact of diversity, equity and inclusion [Internet]. Forbes; 2023 Apr 20 [cited 2025 Feb 13]. Available from: https://www.forbes.com/sites/carolinamilanesi/2023/04/20/the-business-impact-of-diversity-equity-and-inclusion
3. DeMattia A. A mature approach to diversity, equity and inclusion delivers real results [Internet]. Amazon Web Services; 2023 Mar [cited 2025 Feb 13]. Available from: https://aws.amazon.com/executive-insights/content/a-mature-approach-to-diversity-equity-and-inclusion-delivers-real-results/
4. Hinton A Jr, Lambert WM. Moving diversity, equity, and inclusion from opinion to evidence. Cell Rep Med. 2022;3(4):100619. https://doi.org/10.1016/j.xcrm.2022.100619.
5. Averill SL, Pollard JH, Metz CM, DiCamillo PA, Stiles JL, Maiers JJ, Martinez DA, Ferguson N, R Patel A, Zhan X. Grassroots approach to forming a diversity, equity, and inclusion committee in an academic radiology department. Radiographics. 2023;43:e220125. https://doi.org/10.1148/rg.220125.
6. Betancourt JR, Tan-McGrory A, Flores E, López D. Racial and ethnic disparities in radiology: A call to action. J Am Coll Radiol. 2019;16:547–53.
7. Peek ME, Kim KE, Johnson JK, Vela MB. URM candidates are encouraged to apply: a national study to identify effective strategies to enhance racial and ethnic faculty diversity in academic departments of medicine. Acad Med. 2013;88:405–12.
8. Zephyrin LC, Rodriguez J, Rosenbaum S. The case for diversity in the health professions remains powerful [Internet]. The Commonwealth Fund; 2023 July [cited 2025 Feb 13]. Available from: https://www.commonwealthfund.org/blog/2023/case-diversity-health-professions-remains-powerful
9. American Association of Medical Colleges. Underrepresented in Medicine Definition [cited 2025 Feb 13]. Available from: https://www.aamc.org/what-we-do/equity-diversity-inclusion/underrepresented-in-medicine
10. Kelly T, Rodriguez SB. Expanding underrepresented in medicine to include lesbian, gay, bisexual, transgender, and queer individuals. Acad Med. 2022;97:1605–9. https://doi.org/10.1097/ACM.0000000000004720.
11. Page KR, Castillo-Page L, Poll-Hunter N, Garrison G, Wright SM. Assessing the evolving definition of underrepresented minority and its application in academic medicine. Acad Med. 2013;88:67–72. https://doi.org/10.1097/ACM.0b013e318276466c.
12. Perchik JD, Iheke JC, West JT, Smith EN, Milner D, Morgan D, Porter KK. Disruptive behavior: impact on diversity, equity, and inclusion (DEI) in radiology, from the *AJR* special series on DEI. AJR Am J Roentgenol. 2023;221:163–70. https://doi.org/10.2214/AJR.22.28962.
13. Moore R. Trump's executive orders rolling back DEI and accessibility efforts, explained [Internet]. American Civil Liberties Union; 2025 Jan 24 [cited 2025 Feb 13]. Available from: https://www.aclu.org/news/racial-justice/trumps-executive-orders-rolling-back-dei-and-accessibility-efforts-explained
14. Associated Press. These U.S. companies are pulling back on diversity initiatives [Internet]. Time; 2025 Jan 24 [cited 2025 Feb 13]. Available from: https://time.com/7209960/companies-rolling-back-dei/

15. Sherman N. Meta and Amazon scale back diversity initiatives [Internet]. BBC News; 2025 Jan 11 [cited 2025 Feb 13]. Available from: https://www.bbc.com/news/articles/cgmy7xpw3pyo
16. Singer E. Thousands of U.S. government web pages have been taken down since Friday [Internet]. The New York Times; 2025 Feb 2 [cited 2025 Feb 13]. Available from: https://www.nytimes.com/2025/02/02/upshot/trump-government-websites-missing-pages.html
17. Olmsted E. Trump purges information in a terrifying sign of what's coming [Internet]. The New Republic; 2025 Feb 4 [cited 2025 Feb 13]. Available from: https://newrepublic.com/post/191123/donald-trump-purges-information-government-websites
18. Wise J. US health agencies ordered to reinstate webpages removed after Trump's executive order. BMJ. 2025;388:r321. https://doi.org/10.1136/bmj.r321.
19. Perchik JD, Kennedy J, Milner DM, Zarzour JG, Porter KK. Promoting progress and learning from mistakes: results of a radiology department LGBTQ inclusion audit. Acad Radiol. 2022;29:1833–9. https://doi.org/10.1016/j.acra.2022.03.020.
20. Narayan AK, Schaefer PW, Daye D, Alvarez C, Chonde DB, McLoud TC, Flores EJ, Brink JA. Practical tips for creating a diversity, equity, and inclusion committee: experience from a multicenter, academic radiology department. J Am Coll Radiol. 2021;18:1027–37. https://doi.org/10.1016/j.jacr.2021.03.022.
21. Fichera G, Busch IM, Rimondini M, Motta R, Giraudo C. Is empowerment of female radiologists still needed? Findings of a systematic review. Int J Environ Res Public Health. 2021;18:1542. https://doi.org/10.3390/ijerph18041542.
22. Spalluto LB, Arleo EK, Lewis MC, Oates ME, Macura KJ. Addressing needs of women radiologists: opportunities for practice leaders to facilitate change. Radiographics. 2018;38:1626–37. https://doi.org/10.1148/rg.2018180023.
23. Sirtonski L. Wellness, diversity, inclusion key to advancing family leave policies [Internet]. Radiological Society of North America; 2021 Apr 14 [cited 2025 Feb 13]. Available from: https://www.rsna.org/news/2021/april/family-leave-wellness
24. Magudia K, Arleo EK, Porter KK, Ng TSC. A practical guide for paid family and medical leave in radiology, from the *AJR* special series on DEI. AJR Am J Roentgenol. 2023;221:575–81. https://doi.org/10.2214/AJR.23.29327.
25. Mazaheri P, Hawk KE, Ledermann EJ, Lozano KDS, Porter KK. Flexible work arrangements and their impact on women in radiology: RSNA 2021 panel discussion summary sponsored by AAWR and more. Clin Imaging. 2023;94:56–61. https://doi.org/10.1016/j.clinimag.2022.11.012.
26. Lutz A. Radiology technologists working on remote [Internet]. Siemens Healthineers; 2023 Aug 14 [cited 2025 Feb 13]. Available from: https://www.siemens-healthineers.com/perspectives/working-from-home-in-radiology
27. Tso HH, Parikh JR. Mitigating delayed academic promotion of female radiologists due to the COVID pandemic. Clin Imaging. 2021;76:195–8. https://doi.org/10.1016/j.clinimag.2021.04.010.
28. Williams MS, Myers AK, Finuf KD, Patel VH, Marrast LM, Pekmezaris R, Martinez J. Black physicians' experiences with anti-black racism in healthcare systems explored through an attraction-selection-attrition lens. J Bus Psychol. 2023;38:75–88. https://doi.org/10.1007/s10869-022-09825-z.
29. Bredella MA, Fessell D, Thrall JH. Mentorship in academic radiology: why it matters. Insights Imaging. 2019;10:107. https://doi.org/10.1186/s13244-019-0799-2.
30. Sánchez NF, Callahan E, Brewster C, Poll-Hunter N, Sánchez JP. The future LGBT health professional: perspectives on career and personal mentorship. LGBT Health. 2018;5:212–20. https://doi.org/10.1089/lgbt.2017.0134.
31. Harolds JA, Parikh JR, Bluth EI, Dutton SC, Recht MP. Burnout of radiologists: frequency, risk factors, and remedies: a report of the ACR Commission on human resources. J Am Coll Radiol. 2016;13:411–6.
32. Danckers M, Nusynowitz J, Jamneshan L, Shalmiyev R, Diaz R, Radix AE. The sexual and gender minority (LGBTQ+) medical trainee: the journey through medical education. BMC Med Educ. 2024;24:67. https://doi.org/10.1186/s12909-024-05047-4.

33. Gupta Y, Nguyen JK, Shah N, Heitkamp DE, Narayan AK. A National Virtual Mentorship Program in radiology: fostering inclusivity to improve health equity. J Am Coll Radiol. 2022;19:204–6. https://doi.org/10.1016/j.jacr.2021.09.018.
34. Ladd LM, Bonaminio DN, Gonda AS, Gasparis PT, Bell WL, Aaron VD, Heitkamp DE. A mentorship and networking group for women in radiology. J Am Coll Radiol. 2017;14:987–90. https://doi.org/10.1016/j.jacr.2017.01.003.
35. Spalluto LB, Spottswood SE, Deitte LA, Chern A, Dewey CM. A leadership intervention to further the training of female faculty (LIFT-OFF) in radiology. Acad Radiol. 2017;24:709–16. https://doi.org/10.1016/j.acra.2016.12.025.
36. Beanlands RA, Robinson LJ, Venance SL. An LGBTQ+ mentorship program enriched the experience of medical students and physician mentors. Can Med Educ J. 2020;11:e159–62. https://doi.org/10.36834/cmej.69936.
37. Bird A, Zavaletta V, Carroll EF, McGinnis H, Newsome J, Gichoya J, Oakden-Rayner L. Fostering an inclusive workplace for LGBTQIA+ people in radiology and radiation oncology. J Med Imaging Radiat Oncol. 2023;67:193–9. https://doi.org/10.1111/1754-9485.13498.
38. Bonwell CC, Eison JA. Active learning: creating excitement in the classroom. Washington, DC: The George Washington University; 1991.
39. Lavanya KM, Somu LK, Mishra SK. Effectiveness of scenario-based roleplay as a method of teaching soft skills for undergraduate medical students. Int J Appl Basic Med Res. 2024;14:78–84. https://doi.org/10.4103/ijabmr.ijabmr_431_23.
40. University of Brunswick. Creating effective scenarios, case studies and role plays [cited 2025 Feb 13]. Available from: https://www.unb.ca/fredericton/cetl/services/teaching-tips/instructional-methods/creating-effective-scenarios,-case-studies-and-role-plays.html
41. Northern Illinois University Center for Innovative Teaching and Learning. Role playing. In Instructional guide for university faculty and teaching assistants; 2012. [cited 2025 Feb 13]. Available from https://www.niu.edu/citl/resources/guides/instructional-guide
42. University of Wisconsin School of Medicine and Public Health. Department of Radiology. DEI Research and Training. [cited 2025 Feb 13]. Available from: https://radiology.wisc.edu/diversity/research-and-training/
43. Busch IM, Rimondini M, Scott SD, Moretti F, Cecchin D, Wu AW, Giraudo C. Workplace violence in radiology: results of a systematic review. Occup Med (Lond). 2023;73:541–6. https://doi.org/10.1093/occmed/kqad123.
44. Ming JL, Huang HM, Hung SP, Chang CI, Hsu YS, Tzeng YM, Huang HY, Hsu TF. Using simulation training to promote nurses' effective handling of workplace violence: A quasi-experimental study. Int J Environ Res Public Health. 2019;16:3648. https://doi.org/10.3390/ijerph16193648.
45. U.S. Department of Labor. Occupational Safety and Health Administration. Guidelines for preventing workplace violence for healthcare and social service workers; 2016 [cited 2025 Feb 13]. Available from: https://www.osha.gov/sites/default/files/publications/osha3148.pdf
46. University of Michigan Medical School. DEIAJ Curriculum [cited 2025 Feb 13]. Available from: https://medschool.umich.edu/programs-admissions/md-program/md-curriculum/diversity-health-equity/deiaj-curriculum
47. University of South California, Keck School of Medicine. JEDI-WeST [cited 2025 Feb 13]. Available from: https://keck.usc.edu/jedi-west/
48. Andrade Mora DS, Celi Simbaña SS, Simbaña KPC. Mental wellbeing among radiology professionals. Challenges, resilience, and strengths. J Med Imaging Radiat Sci. 2023;54(2S):S115–6. https://doi.org/10.1016/j.jmir.2022.12.007. Epub 2022 Dec 26
49. Bailey CR, Bailey AM, McKenney AS, Weiss CR. Understanding and appreciating burnout in radiologists. Radiographics. 2022;42:E137–9. https://doi.org/10.1148/rg.220037.
50. Camargo A, Radmard M, Dabiri M, Carson KA, Hsu L, Yousem DM. Discrimination faced by radiology residents: an analysis of experiences and mitigation strategies. Curr Probl Diagn Radiol. 2024;53:600–5. https://doi.org/10.1067/j.cpradiol.2024.05.013.

51. Busch IM, Scott SD, Connors C, Story AR, Acharya B, Wu AW. The role of institution-based peer support for health care workers emotionally affected by workplace violence. Jt Comm J Qual Patient Saf. 2021;47:146–56. https://doi.org/10.1016/j.jcjq.2020.11.005.
52. Radiological Society of North America. The Road to addressing equity in Radiology; 2024 Jan 10 [cited 2025 Feb 13]. Available from: https://www.rsna.org/news/2024/january/equity-infographic
53. Lawson MB, Scheel JR, Onega T, Carlos RC, Lee CI. Tackling health disparities in radiology: A practical conceptual framework. J Am Coll Radiol. 2022;19:344–7. https://doi.org/10.1016/j.jacr.2021.09.032.
54. Lopez-Suarez N, Abraham P, Carney M, Castro AA, Narayan AK, Willis M, Spalluto LB, Flores EJ. Practical approaches to advancing health equity in radiology, from the AJR special series on DEI. AJR Am J Roentgenol. 2023;221:7–16. https://doi.org/10.2214/AJR.22.28783.
55. Grimstad FW, Stowell JT, Gaddis M. Survey of experiences of transgender and gender non-binary patients during imaging encounters and opportunities for improvement. AJR Am J Roentgenol. 2020;215:1136–42. https://doi.org/10.2214/AJR.19.22558.
56. Sowinski JS, Gunderman RB. Transgender patients: what radiologists need to know. AJR Am J Roentgenol. 2018;210:1106–10. https://doi.org/10.2214/AJR.17.18904.
57. Radiological Society of North America. RSNA's commitment to diversity, equity and inclusion [cited 2025 Feb 13]. Available from: https://www.rsna.org/about/rsna-diversity-equity-inclusion
58. Radiological Society of North America. Health equity in radiology [cited 2025 Feb 13]. Available from: https://www.rsna.org/practice-tools/radiology-health-equity
59. International Skeletal Society. ISS DEI Webinar Series [cited 2025 Feb 13]. Available from: https://internationalskeletalsociety.com/iss-dei-webinar-series
60. European Society of Radiology. Get to know our committees [cited 2025 Feb 13]. Available from: https://www.myesr.org/about/committees-statutes/
61. Royal College of Radiologists. Equality, Diversity and Inclusion in the RCR. 2022 Jan [cited 2025 Feb 13]. Available from: https://www.rcr.ac.uk/media/qcwh1xpp/2022_equality_diversity_and_inclusion_in_the_rcr_paper.pdf
62. Society of Abdominal Research. Diversity and Inclusion [cited 2025 Feb 13]. Available from: https://abdominalradiology.org/sar-subpages/diversity-and-inclusion-v2/
63. European Society of Breast Imaging. Educational Webinars [cited 2025 Feb 13]. Available from: https://www.eusobi.org/breast-imaging-webinars/
64. International Society for Magnetic Resonance in Medicine. Equity, Diversity, & Inclusion (EDI) [cited 2025 Feb 13]. Available from: https://www.ismrm.org/edi/
65. Radiological Society of North America. Strategic plan [cited 2025 Feb 13]. Available from: https://www.rsna.org/about/reports/strategic-plan
66. Giraudo C, Rosskopf AB, Klauser AS, et al. Gender balance in skeletal radiology: suffrage rather than suffering? Clin Translat Imaging. 2024;12:375–81. https://doi.org/10.1007/s40336-024-00623-6.
67. Bredella MA, Chung CB. Diversity and perception of equity and respect in the Society of Skeletal Radiology (SSR). Skeletal Radiol. 2022;51:849–54. https://doi.org/10.1007/s00256-021-03901-w.
68. Mullen LA, Chu LC, Keen SJ, Macura KJ, Ambinder EB. Lessons learned from a diversity and inclusion survey of the Maryland radiological society. Clin Imaging. 2023;95:56–61. https://doi.org/10.1016/j.clinimag.2022.12.011.
69. Wahab RA, Oluyemi E, Jackson T, Feliciano-Rivera YZ, Roubidoux M, Zhang B, Mehta TS. A needs assessment for inclusion, diversity, and equity: survey results of the society of breast imaging. J Breast Imaging. 2023;5:56–66. https://doi.org/10.1093/jbi/wbac070.
70. Radiology Health Equity Coalition. We see a need to positively impact health care equity in radiology [cited 2025 Feb 13]. Available from: https://www.radhealthequity.org
71. Salem V, McDonagh J, Avis E, Eng PC, Smith S, Murphy KG. Scientific medical conferences can be easily modified to improve female inclusion: a prospective study. Lancet Diabetes Endocrinol. 2021;9:556–9. https://doi.org/10.1016/S2213-8587(21)00177-7.

72. Conley H, Lostis E, MacCormick A, Jenkins P, Gafoor N. Gender representation within radiology conferences in the UK in 2021. Clin Radiol. 2022;77:870–5. https://doi.org/10.1016/j.crad.2022.07.012.
73. HeForShe. United Nations. 2022 [cited 2025 Feb 13]. Available from: https://www.heforshe.org/en
74. Prathivadi Bhayankaram K, Prathivadi Bhayankaram N. Conference panels: do they reflect the diversity of the NHS workforce? BMJ Lead. 2022;6:57–9. https://doi.org/10.1136/leader-2020-000361.
75. The Editors of the Lancet Group. The Lancet Group's commitments to gender equity and diversity. Lancet. 2019;394(10197):452–3. https://doi.org/10.1016/S0140-6736(19)31797-0.
76. University of Washington Medicine, Department of Radiology. Speakers announced for the 2024 Molecular Imaging Symposium [cited 2025 Feb 13]. Available from: https://rad.washington.edu/news/speakers-announced-for-the-2024-molecular-imaging-symposium/
77. Bains A, Osathanugrah P, Sanjiv N, Chiu C, Fiorello MG, Siegel NH, Peeler CE, Distefano AG, Lee HJ, Ness S, Desai MA, Titelbaum JR, Pira T, LaMattina KC, Christiansen SP, Cabral HJ, Subramanian ML. Diverse research teams and underrepresented groups in clinical studies. JAMA Ophthalmol. 2023;141:1037–44. https://doi.org/10.1001/jamaophthalmol.2023.4638.
78. Klontzas ME, Jean J, Turner VL, Balthazar P. Why and how to increase diversity in the radiology trainee workforce. Radiographics. 2022;42:E82–5. https://doi.org/10.1148/rg.220007.
79. DeBenedectis CM, Heitkamp DE, England E, Gaviola GC, Hirsch JA, Ho CP, Jay AK, Kagetsu N, Kalia V, Milburn J, Ong S, Paladin AM, Patel MD, Swanson J, Sarkany DS. A program director's guide to cultivating diversity and inclusion in radiology residency recruitment. Acad Radiol. 2020;27:864–7. https://doi.org/10.1016/j.acra.2019.07.027.
80. Milton AJ, Flores EJ, Charles EF, Elezaby MA, Ward EC, Lee CI, Woods RW, Martin Rother MD, Strigel RM, Narayan AK. Community-based participatory research: A practical guide for radiologists. Radiographics. 2023;43:e220145. https://doi.org/10.1148/rg.220145.
81. Rimondini M, Busch IM, Mazzi MA, Donisi V, Poli A, Bovolenta E, Moretti F. Patient empowerment in risk management: a mixed-method study to explore mental health professionals' perspective. BMC Health Serv Res. 2019;19:382. https://doi.org/10.1186/s12913-019-4215-x.
82. Busch IM, Savazzi S, Bertini G, Cesari P, Guaraldo O, Nosè M, Barbui C, Rimondini M. A practical framework for academics to implement public engagement interventions and measure their impact. Int J Environ Res Public Health. 2022;19:13357. https://doi.org/10.3390/ijerph192013357.
83. European Health Parliament. Patient Empowerment and Centeredness [cited 2025 Feb 13]. Available from: https://www.healthparliament.eu/wp-content/uploads/2017/09/EHP-papers_Patients-empowerment.pdf
84. Náfrádi L, Nakamoto K, Schulz PJ. Is patient empowerment the key to promote adherence? A systematic review of the relationship between self-efficacy, health locus of control and medication adherence. PLoS One. 2017;12:e0186458. https://doi.org/10.1371/journal.pone.0186458.
85. Lauer M, Bernard MA. Analyses of demographic-specific funding rates for Type 1 research project grant and R01-equivalent applications [Internet]. National Institutes of Health, Office of Extramural Research; 2023 Mar 16 [cited 2025 Feb 13]. Available from: https://nexus.od.nih.gov/all/2023/03/16/analyses-of-demographic-specific-funding-rates-for-type-1-research-project-grant-and-r01-equivalent-applications/
86. Abdellatif W, Shao M, Jalal S, Ding J, Vijayasarathi A, Sanelli PC, Castillo M, Norbash A, O'Neill SB, Nicolaou S, Khosa F. Novel geographic thematic study of the largest radiology societies globally: how is gender structure biased within editorial boards? AJR Am J Roentgenol. 2019;213:2–7. https://doi.org/10.2214/AJR.18.20965.
87. Joshi A, Kong W, Yu S, Balasubramanian S, Jankharia B, Agarwal PP. Female representation on radiology journal editorial boards around the world: geographical differences and temporal trends. Acad Radiol. 2022;29:755–62. https://doi.org/10.1016/j.acra.2020.07.004.
88. Piper CL, Scheel JR, Lee CI, Forman HP. Representation of women on radiology journal editorial boards: A 40-year analysis. Acad Radiol. 2018;25:1640–5. https://doi.org/10.1016/j.acra.2018.03.031.

89. White EM, Maduka RC, Ballouz D, Chen H, Wexner SD, Behrns KE, Lillemoe KD, LeMaire SA, Smink DS, Sandhu G. Surgical research journals—under review: an assessment of diversity among editorial boards and outcomes of peer review. Am J Surg. 2021;222:1104–11. https://doi.org/10.1016/j.amjsurg.2021.09.027.
90. American Psychological Association. Bias-Free Language [cited 2025 Feb 13]. Available from: https://apastyle.apa.org/style-grammar-guidelines/bias-free-language
91. American Psychological Association. Inclusive language guide (2nd ed.). 2013 [cited 2025 Feb 13]. Available from: https://www.apa.org/about/apa/equity-diversity-inclusion/language-guidelines.pdf
92. Pal A, Arnet I, Elger BS, Wangmo T. Practices and barriers in developing and disseminating plain-language resources reporting medical research information: A scoping review. Patient. 2024;17:493–518. https://doi.org/10.1007/s40271-024-00700-y.

New Work, Diversity, and Inclusion: Rethinking Radiology for Modern Times

16

Katharina Ronstedt

16.1 Introduction

Why should one place importance on integrating the principles of new work and fostering diversity and inclusion within their service—whether in outpatient care or the hospital environment? While ethical motivations such as fairness and the protection of vulnerable groups are frequently cited, there remain additional, pragmatic advantages, particularly for radiologists carrying the weight of clinical responsibility.

To assess the true necessity of a diverse workforce, it is instructive to apply a practical test: is it possible to fulfill your mission or vision statement in healthcare without the presence of diversity and joint efforts for inclusion? Consider the following generic examples and the pertinent questions they raise:

Vision Statements

- *A healthier future for all*: How can you ensure your efforts embrace "all" members of society—or at the very least, a substantial proportion—without an understanding of which dimensions of diversity are relevant?
- *To become the most trusted healthcare partner*: How will you cultivate trust if your communication cannot be tailored to your patients' varied backgrounds, particularly if you work primarily with colleagues similar to yourself or within rigid hierarchies?
- *Aspiring to lead in improving health and transforming lives*: How meaningful is this ambition if little transformation is reflected within your own workforce?

K. Ronstedt (✉)
Department of Pediatric Radiology, Kassel Hospital GmbH, Kassel, Germany
e-mail: Katharina.Ronstedt@gnh.net

S. Keller-Yamamura, J. Yamamura (eds.), *Inclusive Radiology: Fostering Diversity and Equity in Academic and non-Academic Settings*,
https://doi.org/10.1007/978-3-032-05705-1_16

Mission Statements

- *Providing patient-centered care with outstanding quality, service, and access*: How genuinely patient-centered can your approach be if your staff lack the breadth of personal experience to understand patients' needs?
- *Delivering exemplary healthcare marked by kindness, respect, and dignity*: Can you truly excel if your organizational perspective remains one-dimensional?
- *Striving to enhance the health and well-being of individuals, families, and communities through innovation and excellence*: How can you support those juggling care responsibilities at home if no members of your team can convey firsthand the unique challenges faced during treatment?

If, at any point, the answer to these questions is "I am not certain," it may be time to reflect on the tangible benefits of embracing diversity and new work practices. The advantages are clear: promoting diversity tends to elevate staff satisfaction, encourages creative thinking, and distinguishes proactive leaders from those resistant to change [1, 2].

16.1.1 Brief Ideas About New Work and Its Driving Forces in Radiology

Radiology is entering a period of significant transformation, with urgent workforce shortages now a central concern [3]. Despite efforts to increase training numbers, the supply of new radiologists is not keeping pace with diagnostic and interventional demand, escalating the gap between available professionals and clinical needs [4].

To address this shortage, departments are increasingly opening doors to individuals previously excluded from the workforce—such as those returning from retirement or those with atypical backgrounds—broadening access and supporting diversity within the field [5]. The competition for skilled or educatable radiologists, especially those adaptable to new technologies and working styles, is intensifying as the specialty seeks to attract and retain the best talents [6, 7].

At the same time, the affordability of new imaging technologies, alongside advances in digital safety and clearer legal frameworks for remote and flexible work, is enabling more inclusive and flexible career paths for radiologists [8, 9]. These changes are particularly significant for highly trained professionals whose responsibilities are diversifying both inside and outside the clinical environment.

Another major development is the increasing sub-specialization within radiology [10]. As different pathologies and technologies become more complex, collaboration—both nationally and globally—is essential [11]. This fosters a workforce that values wide-ranging abilities and competences over outdated notions of limitations or organizational barriers.

Overall, radiology's future depends on embracing digital advances, promoting workforce inclusivity, and actively tackling ongoing diversity and equity challenges [12].

16.1.2 New Work Is Not So New: But Today's Challenges Are

The concept of "new work" may sound contemporary, but its foundations are well-established [13]. Throughout history, sustainable work models have succeeded when they balance productivity with personal fulfillment and community connection, for example, The Mondragon Cooperation, founded in 1956, in Basque Country, that makes employees co-owners and emphasizes ongoing education as a major driver of success [14]. What's "new" is not the principle itself, but its modern reinterpretation—updated for present-day technologies, social realities, and workforce expectations [15].

What has truly changed is the level of diversity in today's highly skilled workforce and the range of needs that organizations must now accommodate [16]. This development has been rapidly accelerated by digital innovation, which has made secure, remote work widely accessible. The challenge lies not in recognizing the presence of diversity, but in managing it deliberately and inclusively [17].

Post-COVID, we have a unique opportunity to shift from improvised to intentional diversity strategies. Thanks to growing research across disciplines such as medicine, sociology, and economics [18], we now have both the language and the tools to talk about inclusion, diversity, and the implied organizational needs and define appropriate responses. Institutions can determine which dimensions of diversity they prioritize and evaluate the outcomes of their inclusion efforts for effectiveness and sustainability [1, 19].

Radiology clearly illustrates this shift. As of 2024, around 31% of radiologists in Germany are women [20], 10–15% have direct migration experience, and many more come from families with migration backgrounds [21]. Radiologists with physical disabilities often find the reading room environment comparatively accessible. These realities show why radiology is well positioned to lead by example in applying the principles of new work—adaptive, inclusive, and forward-looking [22].

16.1.3 Core Principles "New Work" and its Implications for Radiology

The term *"new work"* was introduced over 50 years ago by Austrian-American philosopher Frithjof Bergmann [23], who challenged the prevailing economic models that centered exclusively on productivity and wages, often neglecting broader human needs. Bergmann advocated for workplaces where work itself enriches life, empowering individuals to pursue self-determination, autonomy, and personal growth [24]. His vision, originally inspired by automation and the surplus of labor, has grown even more relevant today as technology rapidly reshapes the professional landscape in healthcare [15].

In the modern context, "new work" has evolved into an umbrella term for workplace transformation, prioritizing staff well-being while harnessing the benefits of digitalization, artificial intelligence, and greater mobility. The focus today is on practical, measurable changes that address challenges such as workforce shortages, shifting demographics, and changing employee expectations—issues that resonate strongly within radiology [25].

Though Bergmann's original philosophy may seem utopian, its core principles are highly applicable to radiology, making the field more inclusive and diverse [26]. The essential principles and their implications for radiology are as follows:

1. Autonomy

   Radiology professionals benefit when they have significant control over when and how they work. Flexible scheduling helps those with care responsibilities to better manage competing demands [27].

   Example: Autonomy in scheduling, such as AI-driven shift selection seen at UNC Health, has increased both productivity and satisfaction, offering direct parallels for radiology departments with complex rota needs.
2. Purpose

   Work that is meaningful fosters engagement and resilience [28], especially for staff facing additional barriers [29]. In radiology, this could involve initiatives that remind staff of the importance of their role in patient journeys and well-being, boosting morale and retention.

   Example: Programs that reconnect staff with the human aspects of care—like Sheba Medical Center's "The Heart and Soul of Medicine"—have shown measurable improvements in both patient and staff satisfaction.
3. Flexibility

   Flexibility extends beyond remote work to include adaptable roles and responsibilities, such as job sharing or collaborative leadership. This is vital for supporting clinicians with diverse backgrounds and life situations [30].

   Example: The dyad leadership model in radiology, where responsibility is shared among clinicians, technologists, and administrators, fosters trust, and ensures both clinical and operational priorities are met [31].
4. Collaboration

   Effective teamwork is especially crucial in radiology, a specialty dependent on clear communication across disciplines and departments. Furthermore, effective and well-managed communication enhances job satisfaction and may serve to prevent instances of disruptive behavior among radiology specialists [32], which could otherwise adversely affect both the mental well-being of staff [29] and the overall patient experience [33]. Structured MDT meetings and digital tools enable specialists to contribute regardless of location, making it easier to integrate professionals with varied expertise or backgrounds.

   Example: Online case conferences and cross-institutional MDTs, established during the pandemic, now routinely bring together local and remote subspecialists, highlighting the value of diverse perspectives in clinical decision-making.
5. Lifelong Learning

   Continual education keeps radiologists and teams competitive and engaged, ensuring all can benefit from innovation—regardless of their stage in their career. Providing easy access to ongoing training [34], including upskilling in AI and digital tools, reduces barriers for those new to the specialty or returning after a career break. Furthermore, learning in itself has a positive impact on well-being [35].

Example: The integration of case-based training in the reporting room, on-site lectures, in-person conferences, and remote learning offers many individuals the opportunity to acquire the specific knowledge they require at a given stage in their professional development [36]. *Departments increasingly offer case-based learning platforms and AI workshops tailored to diverse experience levels* [37]. *These resources support junior radiologists in developing core competencies. Furthermore, it helps senior radiologists adapt to new workflows* [38] *while continuing to share their expertise and mentor junior colleagues.*

6. Technology Integration

   Radiology is at the forefront of medical digitalization. By strategically integrating technology and automating routine tasks, teams can focus on complex case interpretation and patient communication [39]. However, it is critical that AI tools are tested for bias and developed with diverse teams in mind, ensuring equitable care for all patient groups [40].

   Example: In 2024, approximately 25% of the publications in "Radiology" *focused on artificial intelligence* [41]*—a testament to its growing importance in the field. Although there are still significant challenges to implementing AI tools in everyday clinical practice, most radiologists express a strong interest in integrating such technologies* [42]. *While concerns about job displacement persist, recent experience has led many opinion leaders to embrace a more balanced view, positioning AI as a supportive rather than a substitutive tool.*

   However, ensuring these new technologies serve all patients equally remains a critical concern—particularly when caring for diverse populations. AI systems are only as good as the data they are trained on, and training datasets often reflect existing inequalities. Underrepresented groups, who frequently face barriers in accessing well-resourced healthcare systems, are rarely represented in high-quality clinical data. In addition, development teams tend to be homogeneous in terms of race, cultural background, and gender, potentially reinforcing hidden biases [40, 43].

   As such, radiology teams that are themselves diverse—and actively advocate for equitable representation—play a vital role in evaluating, adapting, and selecting AI tools that fairly serve all segments of the population. Their engagement is essential to ensuring that technological progress reduces, rather than reinforces, existing disparities in healthcare [5, 44, 45].

7. Work–Life Integration

   Work and personal life are no longer separate spheres—especially in healthcare, where emotional and physical demands are high. The concept of work–life integration recognizes that careers should adapt to the realities of employees' lives, not the other way around [46]. A diverse workforce brings a wide range of personal responsibilities and cultural expectations, which require flexibility and mutual understanding within teams [47].

   Proactively supporting this integration improves staff well-being, reduces burnout, and increases retention across all roles. Structuring policies around shared experience—such as providing reasonable accommodations for pregnancy [48], creating language support systems, or adapting rotas to childcare needs—helps foster a culture of empathy and resilience.

Example: Burnout remains a serious and costly issue in radiology and healthcare. In the United States, it is estimated to create direct costs of over $7600 per doctor per year [49], *not to mention the associated risks of medical errors, declining job performance, and reduced patient satisfaction. Initiatives like individual coaching, on-site wellness programs integrated into staff schedules, or adapting childcare options (such as extending nursery hours or offering emergency cover during overtime shifts)* [30] *have proven effective in reducing toxic stress. These measures not only help retain staff but also support safe, high-quality clinical care* [50].

Implementing more of the other "new work" principles—like flexibility, autonomy, and purpose—further strengthens work–life integration, encouraging a work culture that recognizes people as whole individuals.

16.1.3.1 Implications for Radiology

Embracing these core "new work" principles positions radiology departments to address changing workforce demographics and expectations. By fostering autonomy, purpose, flexibility, collaboration, lifelong learning, smart technology adoption, and genuine work–life integration, radiology can become a blueprint for inclusive and resilient healthcare practice. The field's digital nature and history of innovation make it especially well-suited to lead these changes—delivering benefits not just for staff of all backgrounds and different life circumstances [45, 25], but for the diverse patient populations they serve.

16.1.4 Preparing Radiology Services in Germany for the Future: A Case for Diversity and "New Work"

Germany's healthcare system is undergoing demographic and cultural shifts that demand proactive responses. With an increasingly diverse and international medical trainee population, and evolving expectations around work–life balance and family responsibilities, the structure of traditional clinical work is being challenged. This is particularly urgent in a country where the medical workforce is one of the oldest in Europe [51].

Radiology is uniquely positioned to pioneer new work models in this changing environment and much is already achieved. The next essential step is to intentionally extend these advancements to encompass diversity and inclusion:

- *Remote reporting* is now standard practice in many developed countries and requires limited financial investment to expand.
- *Virtual tumor boards and case discussions* allow for high-level expertise to be shared regardless of physical location, improving clinical decisions without added cost.

- *Workload flexibility* can be achieved by the number of cases assigned to a radiologist. This approach helps prevent burnout and ensures that radiologists can manage their workloads according to their capacity and availability.
- *Data-driven research* is increasingly accessible via PACS and electronic health records, empowering a wider range of professionals to contribute to academic work from anywhere, even from home.
- *Language support from large language models (LLMs)* offers promising solutions for overcoming communication barriers, especially in written reporting.
- *The DRG's diversity network*, now including over 300 members from various diversity dimensions (unpublished data), provides mentorship and connection within and beyond radiology.
- *Radiology's long-standing culture of early technology adoption*, rooted in decades of digital transformation (e.g., analog to PACS), is now part of the professional identity passed on to younger generations.
- *Rapid implementation of AI* and digital tools often leads to immediate time savings and improved clinical quality—outcomes particularly welcome in overstretched departments.

However, not all challenges can—or should—be solved by technological innovation alone. Key elements of a forward-thinking work culture require human-centered attention, especially in a country where medical work force was until recently much standardized in its needs and abilities. What vertical and lateral management shall focus:

- Cultivating a sense of belonging, especially for marginalized professionals.
- Reshaping departmental values to prioritize systematic thinking, creativity, and communication.
- Encouraging genuine curiosity around difference—cultural, cognitive, or experiential—among team members.
- Empowering all team levels, particularly junior staff, to contribute problem-solving ideas and engage in innovation.
- Measuring progress effectively, through thoughtful investment in time, data collection, and analysis.

Ultimately, a thriving radiology department of the future will depend not only on digital tools but on inclusive values, diverse teams, and open-minded leadership.

16.1.5 The Diversity Network of the German Röntgen Society: Lessons Learned from Creating an Inclusive Professional Culture

Founded in 2020, the *Diversity Network of the German Röntgen Society (DRG)* [52] has developed into a dynamic and collaborative platform aimed at promoting diversity, equity, and inclusion (DEI) within the field of radiology. Recognizing the multifaceted nature of professional identity and workplace culture, the Network has structured itself around three primary focus groups: *Women in Radiology*, *Individuals Committed to Inclusion*, and *Radiologists with International Backgrounds*. Each group addresses distinct dimensions of diversity while operating under a cohesive organizational framework.

Importantly, the structure of the Network is intentionally flexible and open-ended. It allows for the formation of additional groups in response to emerging needs, all of which are welcomed and actively supported by the DRG and the Network's coordinators. Regular meetings among elected representatives ensure structured exchanges, foster intergroup collaboration, and facilitate prioritization of pressing diversity-related issues. These processes reinforce collective learning and accountability while aligning closely with the strategic aims of the DRG.

The Network's experience so far offers valuable insights that may serve as a practical reference for *senior medical leaders and innovative young radiologists* seeking to embed diversity in their own institutions. Rather than offering an abstract framework, we hope to provide practice-based model for establishing inclusive systems within challenging clinical environments.

16.1.5.1 Valuing the Perspectives of Non-Leadership Staff

An essential principle guiding the Network's efforts has been the recognition that sustainable diversity initiatives must incorporate the experiences of staff who do not currently occupy formal leadership positions. These individuals often face the most structural barriers yet remain underrepresented in organizational decision-making.

Take, for example, the situation of women in radiology—particularly mothers of more than one child—whose career trajectories are often disrupted not solely due to pregnancies and part-time work [53], but due to the cumulative effect of diminished research output during periods of family responsibility. Given that academic advancement remains closely tied to publication quantity and visibility [54], this group is frequently excluded from traditional paths to leadership. Moreover, a lack of familiarity with assertive behavioral norms within hierarchical systems may further marginalize their input.

The Network has actively created space for these perspectives to surface, particularly through small-group sessions and informal discussions. Breaking away from overly structured formats has enabled broader participation and allowed for the emergence of themes otherwise underexplored in more traditional settings. These insights are then synthesized and fed back into wider forums, creating a feedback loop that values both grassroots input and strategic alignment.

16.1.5.2 Creating Inclusive Spaces for Dialogue

Safe and accessible environments for discussion are particularly important for members of the radiological community who may feel uncertain. Among these are early-career professionals who have migrated to Germany and are in the early stages of adapting to their new professional landscape.

Initial reluctance among this group to participate in discussions was often found to stem not from lack of expertise but from language barriers—whether real, perceived, or culturally embedded. The Network responded by creating explicitly welcoming spaces and by validating the unique lived experiences these professionals bring. Their input proved to be not only insightful but indispensable in designing responsive, peer-informed solutions.

16.1.5.3 Recognizing the Work Behind the Work

Diversity and inclusion efforts, might it be in a broader network or in a local hospital, usually require time and energy in addition to existing professional responsibilities. Many members of the Network contribute alongside clinical duties, research obligations, or family responsibilities. Recognizing this additional commitment is both ethically necessary and strategically effective.

The DRG has played a commendable role in supporting these efforts, taking responsibility for administrative coordination, providing technological infrastructure, and facilitating access to decision-makers when needed. These structural supports signal institutional acknowledgment and validation, which fosters motivation and long-term engagement among active contributors.

16.1.5.4 Drawing Strength from Diversity Within and Across Diversity Dimensions

One of the Network's distinctive features is its commitment to diversity across multiple dimensions, not limited to gender, ethnicity, or nationality. Equally valued are differences in career stage, professional experience, and disciplinary orientation. Focus groups typically include early-career radiologists, mid-career academics, and established consultants—all united by a shared commitment to positive transformation.

Success, however, relies not only on bringing together a diverse group but also on identifying shared values and goals. Each group's focus naturally offers a foundation for collective purpose. At the broader Network level, strategic alignment is fostered through the expression of common principles: Supporting one dimension of diversity often encourages solidarity and action across others, reinforcing a culture of inclusion. For example, advocating for parenting colleagues often extends to supporting those with other caregiving responsibilities; promoting language access uplifts immigrant professionals; and inclusive leadership strengthens the organization as a whole. As one member aptly stated, "It does not matter from which side we cut the cake of diversity—as long as it ends up on the table of those who shape the future."

16.1.5.5 Leadership Support

Efforts to embed diversity within clinical and academic institutions must be supported by leadership engagement. While bottom-up energy is crucial, long-term success hinges on the ability to establish trusting relationships with boards, department heads, and other senior figures.

The Network has made a conscious effort to avoid polarizing language or oppositional dynamics from the start. Instead, it emphasizes the shared mission and mutual respect that exists between diversity advocates and institutional leaders.

Acknowledging the wisdom, managerial competence, and professional commitment of organizational leadership has helped the Network build credibility and elicit strong and sustained support.

16.1.5.6 Lowering the Barriers to Entry

To guarantee long-term momentum, the Network has prioritized ease of access to ensure new members can join and engage without undue pressure. Communication takes place through a commonly used messaging app, and participation begins with a simple self-introduction and a shared portrait. This balance of professionalism and informality fosters accessibility without compromising on standards.

Notably, incidents of negative or disruptive behavior have been virtually nonexistent—a surprising outcome given the open nature of the forum. This may be due in part to the relatively tight-knit radiology community in Germany, where professional reputation remains a strong regulating force. Nevertheless, this success also speaks to the Network's effective tone and culture of mutual respect.

16.1.5.7 Managing Internal Dynamics and Competing Priorities

As in any multifaceted initiative, occasional tensions can arise within diversity efforts—particularly around resource allocation or levels of visibility. Representatives from various focus groups are often highly attuned to one another's challenges yet may, at times, experience a sense of competition or inequity.

In anticipation of such complications, the Network has implemented several strategies, including

- Emphasizing individuals' intersectional identities and overlapping experiences
- Promoting active social and professional connections across focus groups to build camaraderie
- Advocating for sufficient resources to avoid perceptions of scarcity
- Consulting experienced board members and staff at the DRG's headquarters whose institutional memory and problem-solving acumen prove invaluable

It is our hope that the insights and experiences drawn from the Network's journey will offer meaningful guidance to those who are committed to fostering greater equity and inclusion within their own organizations. The lessons we have learned—through both success and constructive friction—may provide a useful foundation or source of inspiration for or all those striving to build inclusive, high-performing radiology entities in an increasingly complex clinical world.

Bibliography

1. Kochan T, Bezrukova K, Ely R, et al. The effects of diversity on business performance: report of the diversity research network. Hum Resour Manag. 2003;42(1):3–21. https://doi.org/10.1002/hrm.10061.

2. van Knippenberg D, Haslam SA, Platow MJ. Unity through diversity: value-in-diversity beliefs, work group diversity, and group identification. Group Dyn Theory Res Pract. 2007;11(3):207–22. https://doi.org/10.1037/1089-2699.11.3.207.
3. Bender CE, Bansal S, Wolfman D, Parikh JR. 2019 ACR commission on human resources workforce survey. J Am Coll Radiol. 2020;17(5):673–5. https://doi.org/10.1016/j.jacr.2020.01.012.
4. Jeganathan S. The growing problem of radiologist shortages: Australia and New Zealand's perspective. Korean J Radiol. 2023;24(11):1043. https://doi.org/10.3348/kjr.2023.0831.
5. Lightfoote JB, Fielding JR, Deville C, et al. Improving diversity, inclusion, and representation in radiology and radiation oncology part 1: why these matter. J Am Coll Radiol. 2014;11(7):673–80. https://doi.org/10.1016/j.jacr.2014.03.007.
6. Jing AB, Garg N, Zhang J, Brown JJ, Mcwilliams B. AI solutions to the radiology workforce shortage. npj Health Syst. 2025;2(1):1–6. https://doi.org/10.1038/s44401-025-00023-6.
7. Afshari Mirak S, Harsha Tirumani S, Ramaiya N, Mohamed I. The growing nationwide radiologist shortage: current opportunities and ongoing challenges for international medical graduate radiologists. Radiology. 2025;314(3) https://doi.org/10.1148/RADIOL.232625/ASSET/IMAGES/LARGE/RADIOL.232625.VA.JPEG.
8. Kwee TC, Kwee RM. Workload of diagnostic radiologists in the foreseeable future based on recent (2024) scientific advances: updated growth expectations. Eur J Radiol. 2025;187:112103. https://doi.org/10.1016/J.EJRAD.2025.112103.
9. Kelly BS, Quinn C, Belton N, Lawlor A, Killeen RP, Burrell J. Cybersecurity considerations for radiology departments involved with artificial intelligence. Eur Radiol. 2023;33(12):8833–41. https://doi.org/10.1007/s00330-023-09860-1.
10. Rupreht M, Ricci P, Prosch H, Adriaensen MEAPM. Subspecialisation in radiology in Europe, a survey of the accreditation council of imaging. Insights Imaging. 2023;14(1):159. https://doi.org/10.1186/S13244-023-01481-Y.
11. Dewey M, Bosserdt M, Dodd JD, Thun S, Kressel HY. Clinical imaging research: higher evidence, global collaboration, improved reporting, and data sharing are the grand challenges. Radiology. 2019;291(3):547–52. https://doi.org/10.1148/RADIOL.2019181796.
12. Becker M. How to prepare for a bright future of radiology in Europe. Insights Imaging. 2023;14(1):1–8. https://doi.org/10.1186/S13244-023-01525-3/.
13. Stafford K, Duncan KA, Dane S, Winter M. A research model of sustainable family businesses. Fam Bus Rev. 1999;12(3):197–208. https://doi.org/10.1111/J.1741-6248.1999.00197.X.
14. Morlà-Folch T, Aubert Simon A, de Freitas AB, Hernández-Lara AB. The Mondragon case: companies addressing social impact and dialogic methodologies. Int J Qual Methods. 2021:20. https://doi.org/10.1177/16094069211058614.
15. Werther S, Brenning S. New Work – ein konzeptioneller Überblick. New Work, Leadership und Human Resources Management im Tourismus. Published online 2024. p. 3–22. https://doi.org/10.1007/978-3-658-42932-4_1.
16. Anand R, Winters MF. A retrospective view of corporate diversity training from 1964 to the present. Acad Manage Learn Educ. 2008;7(3):356–72. https://doi.org/10.5465/AMLE.2008.34251673.
17. Liu J, Zhu Y, Wang H. Managing the negative impact of workforce diversity: the important roles of inclusive HRM and employee learning-oriented behaviors. Front Psychol. 2023;14:1117690. https://doi.org/10.3389/FPSYG.2023.1117690/BIBTEX.
18. Ashikali T, Groeneveld S, Kuipers B. The role of inclusive leadership in supporting an inclusive climate in diverse public sector teams. Rev Publ Pers Adm. 2021;41(3):497–519. https://doi.org/10.1177/0734371X19899722.
19. Allen RS, Dawson G, Wheatley K, White CS. Perceived diversity and organizational performance. Empl Relat. 2008;30(1):20–33. https://doi.org/10.1108/01425450810835392.
20. Ärztestatistik zum 31. Dezember 2024 Bundesgebiet gesamt. https://wwwbundesaerztekammerde/fileadmin/user_upload/BAEK/Ueber_uns/Statistik/AErztestatistik_2024pdf. Accessed 15 July 2025.
21. 2023 - Bundesärztekammer. Accessed 15 July 2025. https://www.bundesaerztekammer.de/baek/ueber-uns/aerztestatistik/2023.

22. Shore LM, Cleveland JN, Sanchez D. Inclusive workplaces: a review and model. Hum Resour Manag Rev. 2018;28(2):176–89. https://doi.org/10.1016/J.HRMR.2017.07.003.
23. Frithjof Bergmann—Frithjof Bergmann - New Work New Culture. Accessed 21 July 2025. https://newwork-newculture.dev/frithjofbergmann/.
24. Autor D, Chin C, Salomons A, Seegmiller B. New frontiers: the origins and content of new work, 1940–2018. Q J Econ. 2024;139(3):1399–465. https://doi.org/10.1093/QJE/QJAE008.
25. Chekmeyan M, DeBenedectis CM. Diversity, equity, and inclusion programs in radiology: data-driven strategies for success, from the AJR special series on DEI. Am J Roentgenol. 2023;220(6):780–6. https://doi.org/10.2214/AJR.22.28422.
26. Stiglbauer B, Penz M, Batinic B. Work values across generations: development of the New Work Values Scale (NWVS) and examination of generational differences. Front Psychol. 2022;13:1028072. https://doi.org/10.3389/FPSYG.2022.1028072.
27. Belfi LM, Retrouvey M, Alexandre Frigini L, et al. Current trends in remote and flexible work options in radiology and perception of impact on radiologist well-being. Acad Radiol. 2025;32(3):1661–70. https://doi.org/10.1016/J.ACRA.2024.11.071.
28. Nair AK, Adluru N, Finley AJ, et al. Purpose in life as a resilience factor for brain health: diffusion MRI findings from the midlife in the U.S. study. Front Psychiatry. 2024;15:1355998. https://doi.org/10.3389/FPSYT.2024.1355998.
29. Bailey CR, Bailey AM, McKenney AS, Weiss CR. Understanding and appreciating burnout in radiologists. Radiographics. 2022;42(5):E137–9. https://doi.org/10.1148/RG.220037.
30. Spalluto LB, Arleo EK, Lewis MC, Oates ME, Macura KJ. Addressing needs of women radiologists: opportunities for practice leaders to facilitate change. Radiographics. 2018;38(5):1626–37. https://doi.org/10.1148/RG.2018180023.
31. Saxena A. Challenges and success strategies for dyad leadership model in healthcare. Healthc Manage Forum. 2021;34(3):137–48. https://doi.org/10.1177/0840470420961522.
32. Ulreich S, Harris RD, Sze G, Moriarity AK, Bluth E. The disruptive radiologist. J Am Coll Radiol. 2015;12(8):800–4. https://doi.org/10.1016/J.JACR.2015.02.013.
33. Pearce CL. The future of leadership: combining vertical and shared leadership to transform knowledge work. Acad Manag Exec. 2004;18(1):47–57. https://doi.org/10.5465/AME.2004.12690298.
34. Nguyen XV, Adams SJ, Hobbs SK, Ganeshan D, Wasnik AP. Radiologist as lifelong learner: strategies for ongoing education. Acad Radiol. 2019;26(8):1120–6. https://doi.org/10.1016/J.ACRA.2019.03.019.
35. Brashovetska O, Brehm S. Does learning equal happiness? Research-based evidence on the impact of lifelong learning on subjective well-being. Published online 2023. Accessed 20 July 2025. https://lup.lub.lu.se/luur/download?func=downloadFile&recordOId=9115278&fileOId=9115279.
36. Adriaensen M, Ricci P, Prosch H, Rupreht M. Evolution of continuing medical education in radiology: on-site vs remote. Insights Imaging. 2024;15(1):192. https://doi.org/10.1186/S13244-024-01764-Y.
37. Vásquez A, Palazuelos G, Pinzon BA, Romero J. Blended learning in radiology: evaluation of a nationwide training program on breast imaging. J Am Coll Radiol. 2018;15(3):458–62. https://doi.org/10.1016/J.JACR.2017.11.008.
38. Chetty K. AI literacy for an ageing workforce: leveraging the experience of older workers. OBM Geriatrics. 2023;7(3):1–17. https://doi.org/10.21926/OBM.GERIATR.2303243.
39. Najjar R. Redefining radiology: a review of artificial intelligence integration in medical imaging. Diagnostics. 2023;13(17):2760. https://doi.org/10.3390/DIAGNOSTICS13172760.
40. Hilling DE, Ihaddouchen I, Buijsman S, Townsend R, Gommers D, van Genderen ME. The imperative of diversity and equity for the adoption of responsible AI in healthcare. Front Artif Intell. 2025;8:1577529. https://doi.org/10.3389/FRAI.2025.1577529.
41. Moy L. Top publications in radiology, 2024. Radiology. 2024;313(3) https://doi.org/10.1148/RADIOL.243436.

42. Cancela J, Roche S, Wittal CG, et al. Physicians' attitudes and acceptance towards artificial intelligence in medical care: a qualitative study in Germany. Front Digit Health. 2025;7:1616827. https://doi.org/10.3389/FDGTH.2025.1616827.
43. Why Diversity in AI Matters: Moving towards inclusivity and away from bias - Artificial intelligence. Accessed 20 July 2025. https://nationalcentreforai.jiscinvolve.org/wp/2025/06/30/why-diversity-in-ai-matters-moving-towards-inclusivity-and-away-from-bias/.
44. Gomez LE, Bernet P. Diversity improves performance and outcomes. J Natl Med Assoc. 2019;111(4):383–92. https://doi.org/10.1016/J.JNMA.2019.01.006.
45. Chapman CH, Hwang WT, Both S, Thomas CR, Deville C. Current status of diversity by race, hispanic ethnicity, and sex in diagnostic radiology. Radiology. 2014;270(1):232–40. https://doi.org/10.1148/RADIOL.13130101.
46. Wei JL, Villwock JA. Balance versus integration: work-life considerations. Otolaryngol Clin N Am. 2021;54(4):823. https://doi.org/10.1016/J.OTC.2021.05.007.
47. Schmidt M, Steigenberger N, Berndtzon M, Uman T. Cultural diversity in health care teams: a systematic integrative review and research agenda. Health Care Manag Rev. 2023;48(4):311–22. https://doi.org/10.1097/HMR.0000000000000379.
48. Seely JM. Women in radiology: challenges and opportunities. J Breast Imag. 2024;6(5):539–46. https://doi.org/10.1093/JBI/WBAE030.
49. Doctor burnout costs health care system $4.6 billion a year, Harvard study says — Harvard Gazette. Accessed 20 July 2025. https://news.harvard.edu/gazette/story/2019/07/doctor-burnout-costs-health-care-system-4-6-billion-a-year-harvard-study-says/.
50. Large-scale European study into preventing burnout due to stress among staff in and around the operating theater. Accessed 20 July 2025. https://medicalxpress.com/news/2024-07-large-scale-european-burnout-due.html.
51. [hlth_rs_phys] Physicians by sex and age. Accessed 15 July 2025. https://ec.europa.eu/eurostat/databrowser/view/hlth_rs_phys/default/table?lang=en.
52. Das Netzwerk | Accessed 22 July 2025. https://www.diversity.drg.de/de-DE/7019/das-netzwerk/.
53. Song J, Cheng TC. How do gender differences in family responsibilities affect doctors' labour supply? Evidence from Australian panel data. Soc Sci Med. 2020;265:113475. https://doi.org/10.1016/J.SOCSCIMED.2020.113475.
54. Buddeberg-Fischer B, Stamm M, Buddeberg C, et al. The impact of gender and parenthood on physicians' careers - professional and personal situation seven years after graduation. BMC Health Serv Res. 2010;10:40. https://doi.org/10.1186/1472-6963-10-40.

Parenting and Motherhood in Academic and Clinical Medicine

17

Eva See

17.1 Impacts of Pregnancy and Motherhood on Mother Physicians

The increasing proportion of women in medical schools, now exceeding 50% of graduates, has brought the (lack of) compatibility of motherhood and medical careers into focus. Despite this shift, traditional gender roles persist, with women bearing a disproportionate burden of domestic and caregiving responsibilities [1]. The COVID-19 pandemic starkly highlighted these disparities, as evidenced by a significant decline in publications by female scientists [2]. This trend underscores the impact of childcare disruptions and increased unpaid care work on women's professional productivity [1, 2].

Structural and institutional barriers within the medical profession continue to disadvantage women during pregnancy and (early) motherhood, particularly during critical career stages. Inadequate workplace policies and lack of supportive mechanisms contribute to this disparity, often exacerbated by supervisors' insufficient knowledge or unwillingness to accommodate, relegating (expectant) mothers to career paths with fewer opportunities for advancement. These setbacks manifest in slower progress toward specialist status, reduced research output, and limited access to leadership roles, further entrenching gender disparities in academic and clinical medicine [2].

The difficulties in achieving work–life integration and inadequate support for maternity/parental leave and return-to-work can lead to career dissatisfaction among physician mothers [3]. The concerns over family and medical career (im-)balance

E. See (✉)
Department of Radiology, Hochwaldkrankenhaus Bad Nauheim - Gesundheitszentrum Wetterau gGmbH, Bad Nauheim, Germany
e-mail: eva.see@gz-wetterau.de

S. Keller-Yamamura, J. Yamamura (eds.), *Inclusive Radiology: Fostering Diversity and Equity in Academic and non-Academic Settings*,
https://doi.org/10.1007/978-3-032-05705-1_17

have been associated with high rates of burnout among female physicians [4]. As the demand for qualified physicians grows due to demographic changes and skilled worker shortages, it is crucial to foster a family-friendly workplace culture, adapting structures to modern family needs easing time management between professional duties, family responsibilities, and further preferences for personal well-being [5–8]. This adaptation would enable more parents to pursue a medical career without neglecting their families and health.

Especially fathers noticeably participating in care work and other family responsibilities may experience similar circumstances; however, mothers face additional challenges that are gender-specific. These include discrimination at work (long) before and during pregnancy, including deficient responses to adverse outcomes such as miscarriages, as well as during and after maternity/parental leave. (Potential) motherhood, with mothers typically/naturally being the primary attachment figure in early childhood [1, 2], remains a stigma in health economics analogous to what Claudia Goldin defines as "greedy work": jobs that disproportionately reward longer hours or less flexible schedules, paying more per hour when employees work extended hours or have less control over their time. She argues that this structure of work is at the heart of gender pay disparities, as it often forces women to choose between career advancement and family responsibilities, perpetuating inequality in the workplace [9]. This chapter aims to show ways to improve the compatibility of paid employment and unpaid care work for parents in academic and clinical medicine, with a focus on physician mothers.

17.2 Key Factors of a Necessary Structural Change

Recommendations for Improving Work-Life Integration and Career Support of Mother Physicians in Clinical and Academic Context

Demographic change, shortage of skilled workers, and the increasing feminization of the medical workforce have brought the issues mentioned above to the forefront. They highlight the demand of physicians of all educational levels and the consequent need for systemic changes in the medical profession in order to support physicians who are also parents or wish to become parents. In order to meet the nationally required workforce and keep up with the international labor market, it is necessary that parent physicians have the opportunity to contribute to general care, undergo and complete specialist training, gain the status of specialist physicians, and develop their careers in both academic and clinical medicine. In order to empower parents in medicine to accomplish these goals, it is important to adapt structures to the needs of a modern family life with shared unpaid care work and paid employment—not only enabling work, but also enabling healthy families embedded in an appreciative supportive work environment [8].

Here are some of the most important recommendations for the supportive policies needed for a cultural shift in academic and clinical medicine in order to better support physician parents based on current research and a modern Zeitgeist.

17.2.1 Facing Discrimination and Bias with a Supportive Environment

Success depends on private support, childcare availability, and workplace backing from colleagues, supervisors, and management. Collegial consideration and open communication foster positive environments, particularly for pregnant staff or those returning from parental leave. Leaders should implement a family-friendly environment and acknowledge contributions from parents, emphasizing their value despite their family obligations. These measures contribute to their long-term career, family success, and satisfaction. The following is needed to address and eliminate maternity discrimination in the workplace [6, 7, 10–12]:

- Implement policies that do not perpetuate gender and sexual orientation-based inequalities.
- Foster an institutional culture that normalizes conversations about parenting and work–life (im-)balance, reducing stigma associated with parental responsibilities and other care work.
- Implement policies that support both parents in sharing childcare responsibilities, promoting equal involvement.
- Train supervisors to recognize and support the unique challenges faced by physician parents, promoting equity in evaluations and career advancement.
- Encourage open communication between supervisors and working parents to address challenges and find solutions.
- Acknowledge feasible professional commitment during different stages of parenthood.
- Appreciate particularly vulnerable employees such as pregnant woman, mother physicians early after childbirth and during/after breastfeeding as important employees, who take on numerous tasks in various areas, thus providing significant support to employers and co-workers.

17.2.2 Mentoring Networks

Colleagues and mentors play a crucial role in supporting parents in medicine by helping to navigate the challenges of balancing their paid work with family responsibilities throughout their medical careers. An effective mentorship can enhance career advancement and improve strategies for better work–life integration, therefore increasing satisfaction in both professional and personal roles [8, 13]. Mentoring can take place as professional support in areas such as career guidance, skill development and networking opportunities [14], as well as personal support, including strategies for a functioning compatibility of paid employment and family life (including both unpaid care work and quality time), emotional support, and creating flexible work arrangements [15]. What to consider [6, 16]:

- Implement structured mentorship programs tailored for parent physicians, combined with other mentoring programs (e.g., for professional development).
- Have mentees pair early in their careers or specialty training with mentors (e.g., experienced mother/father physicians) who have successfully navigated similar challenges.
- Provide access to parenting resources, workshops, coaching, and support groups [e.g., employee resource groups (ERGs)] to share experiences, advice, and resources in order to help working parents develop effective strategies.
- Unite diverse networks of physicians for improved work–life integration.

17.2.3 Specialty Choice

The anticipation of childbearing affects female physicians' specialty choices, with some opting for (perceived) less-demanding specialties to better reconcile paid employment and family life [4]. Others switch their specialties during training, adding up to the overall time needed in order to become a specialist. Integrating discussions about family planning, compatibility, and well-being into medical education and specialty training can better prepare future physicians and residents for the challenges of parenting in medicine [17]. This can include guidance on fertility, pregnancy, and childcare, as well as career options. Addressing typical gender-/family-specific topics and pitfalls early in medical education and specialty training may enable young medical students and physicians to make more informed decisions about their professional future based on their individual goals and focus.

Here are the key factors that might especially influence parent physicians and those wishing to become parents in their specialty choice:

- Flexible work hours and predictable schedules ease childcare planning, allowing for a better compatibility of paid employment and family life, which then increases overall well-being.
- Opportunities for part-time work or shared schedules, therefore providing more options for balancing career and family responsibilities.
- Lower frequency of on-call duties and emergencies, consequently reducing disruptions to personal and family time.
- Regular office hours with minimal night shifts to contribute to a more stable home life and consistent presence for children.
- Potential for practice-based work, hence offering greater control over scheduling and work environment, making it easier to accommodate family needs.

17.2.4 Specialty Training

The skilled worker shortage emphasizes the importance of a swift progress to specialist status. This need can be met by training networks (hospital–hospital, hospital–practice, practice–practice) with smart rotation plans flexible enough to respond positively in cases of shortages in staff [5]. Maintaining professional roles for parents and parents-to-be during the time of their specialty training sustains skills and competence. The following lists out ways to provide support for women with children, who are particularly affected by work–life (im-)balance issues [18], by enabling continued training and facilitating progress toward specialist status [5, 12, 19–24]:

- Foster an institutional culture that normalizes continued specialty training during pregnancy, after maternal/parental leave, and throughout parenthood.
- Standardize a nationwide 38-hour week as a full-time equivalent in credit for specialty training, and credit working over 100% on the annual balance to the period of specialty training, taking into account shifts and overtime.
- Implement nationwide flexible part-time models crediting at least 20% of the full-time equivalent for specialty training.
- Offer shared rotations.
- Implement positive interpretations of maternity protection laws.
- Introduce standardized risk assessments for all workplaces and execute changes needed in order to ensure continued specialty training during pregnancy and lactation period, expressly also in challenging areas (e.g., control or monitoring areas, operating room).
- Upon notification of pregnancy, offer a conversation with the pregnant physician and their supervisor/employer in which the previous training content, including a rotation plan and career development, is laid out and a structured plan for the continuation of their specialty training and career path during and after pregnancy, maternity leave and, if applicable, parental leave is setup.
- Use positive job lists from professional societies and associations aiding their implementation.
- Utilize the opportunity to hire retired specialists as freelancers to take over shifts in the afternoon and evening for regular workload and supervise/teach physicians in specialty training.

17.2.5 Work Integration

Parent physicians, especially mothers, often cease full-time employment due to difficulties balancing their medical career with parenthood [4, 25]. Fostering the following strategies toward a more modern, flexible institutional culture might increase their work integration while being beneficial for all employees [5, 6, 9–12, 16, 18, 23, 24]:

- Promote compatibility of paid employment and other individual aspects of life, such as family responsibilities and further preferences for personal well-being, as a priority for all healthcare professionals.

- Create a family-friendly workplace culture that values a functioning compatibility of paid employment and family life (including both unpaid care work and quality time), supporting parents' needs and well-being.
- Standardize adaptable full- and part-time work arrangements and (top) job-sharing options with flexible scheduling and adjustable work hours, as well as remote work options without penalizing career advancement opportunities.
- Promote equitable clinical duty coverage without straining colleagues, including training more employees at the same skill level and utilizing the opportunity to hire retired specialists as freelancers to take over shifts in the afternoon and evening for regular workload and supervise/teach physicians in specialty training.
- Create ideal positions that offer long-term prospects for committed individuals recognizing their individual contributions to the institution.
- Long-term staff retention increases the quality of the company through employees with many years of experience.

Supporting participation through childcare options [5, 8, 10, 23]:

- Expand childcare nationwide, also suitable for those working shift systems.
- Provide on-site childcare facilities or subsidized access to local childcare services to alleviate logistical challenges, including those due to regular working hours and especially for physicians working nonstandard hours.
- Develop emergency childcare/backup care options, including entitlement to emergency child care in all kindergartens, to address sudden scheduling conflicts, especially during on-call shifts, sick leave covers, or other unexpected situations.
- Collaborate with childcare providers, including au pair agencies, to offer discounted or convenient care options for employees.

Acknowledging potential impact on parents' health [10, 18]:

- Foster an institutional culture that normalizes parenthood without straining colleagues, accepting that the parental workforce can be diminished (e.g., due to chronic lack of sleep, absent days due to sickness or children's holidays), therefore increasing the workload of the colleagues present.
- Address the disproportionate impact of work hours on female physicians' burnout rates.

17.2.6 Career Support

Pregnancy and motherhood can affect the long-term career plans of mother physicians, potentially altering their professional goals and aspirations [4]. They often experience fewer career opportunities and are less likely to be encouraged to pursue leadership roles [26]. Career advancement may be slowed additionally by turning down professional opportunities, leadership roles, and scholarship options due to (perceived) lack of compatibility of work and family responsibilities [27]. The difficulties in achieving work–life integration and inadequate support for maternity leave and return-to-work can lead to career dissatisfaction among physician mothers [3].

Supporting parent physicians, especially mothers, in their career broadens skill availability and improves career prospects for all employees. Recommendations include [5, 6, 12, 16, 23, 24]:

- Increase career flexibility, including medical/specialty training and work as a specialist, therefore decreasing career disruptions.
- Create targeted career development programs for mother physicians, thereby addressing and eliminating the unique challenges they face in balancing family and career aspirations.
- Provide leadership training and opportunities specifically for mother/parent physicians to ensure their representation in decision-making roles.
- Promote shared leadership models, enabling parents to hold senior positions without full-time burdens.
- Create positions adaptable to personal life trajectories, considering individual specialization, qualifications, and preferences.
- Support the achievement of subspecialties or special competencies.

17.2.7 Academic Pathway

The challenges of balancing motherhood and a medical career may affect long-term research output and academic advancement negatively [4]. Measures to support parent physicians to pursue an academic pathway successfully [5, 16, 19, 28–30]:

- Foster close cooperation between academic institutions, policymakers, and clinician scientists.
- Boost university medicine as a key player in both research and healthcare systems.
- Create advocacy committees within academic institutions to address systemic biases and promote gender equity.
- Implement science-oriented human resource programs tailored to clinician scientists' needs, balancing individual requirements with those of the institution.
- Introduce grant extensions and flexible deadlines for researchers who take parental leave, ensuring continuity in academic productivity.
- Develop and implement metrics that recognize the quality of research output rather than solely the quantity, particularly during periods of caregiving.
- Create more flexible career paths for clinician scientists, including mother physicians, such as developing varied career models in university medicine and positions adaptable to personal life trajectories, considering individual specialization, qualifications, and preferences, as well as taking into account specific location needs.

- Create positions that offer long-term prospects for committed individuals.
- Recognize individual contributions to the institution.
- Narrow the salary gap between academic and nonacademic radiologists.
- Standardize a nationwide 38-hour week as a full-time equivalent in credit for specialty training, and credit working over 100% on the annual balance to the period of specialty training, taking into account shifts and overtime.
- Credit research periods proportionately to the time period of specialty training.

17.2.8 Family Planning and Pregnancy

Women physicians report delay in starting a family to attain specific career milestones or choosing specialties based on perceived family-friendliness [7], which can impact their overall career trajectory [26]. A delayed childbearing age and demanding daily physician duties may result in increased infertility rates and adverse pregnancy outcomes [7].

How family planning can be addressed [10, 17, 31]:

- Offer transparent information and mentorship during medical education and throughout specialty training, normalizing open family planning, and addressing fear of negative effects on medical education, specialty training, and furthering their career.
- Take measures facing the 1 in 4 female physicians experiencing infertility by implementing policies that support fertility treatment, adoption, and foster care.

How pregnant physicians can be supported:

Comprehensive structural changes are needed to enable self-determined individual decisions, according to the motto: "everything can, nothing has to."Based on this, a trusting working environment is a prerequisite for enabling open, honest discussions about the possibilities and conditions of continued work and specialty training, in which the pregnant physician can express any concerns and wishes. Overall premise for continued work is the physical and mental well-being of the pregnant or breastfeeding physician and a healthy (unborn) baby. Thus, continued employment during pregnancy and breastfeeding must be desired by the (expectant) mother. Flexibility and the willingness to deal with changes of the workplace are needed on both sides [12]. What is recommended [5, 8, 10, 12, 21, 23, 24]:

- Foster an institutional culture that normalizes continued work in accordance to maternity laws (e.g., clinical duty coverage), as well as absent days during pregnancy and parenthood, highlighting the overall support and relief of colleagues through the continued work of the (expectant) mother.
- Implement positive interpretations of maternity protection laws.
- Appoint a maternity protection officer, who may receive reports from pregnant physicians, offering advice and support to them and, if necessary, acts as a mod-

erator between the pregnant or breastfeeding physician and the employer, supervisor, and occupational physician. She is to be subject to confidentiality.

- Introduce standardized risk assessments of all workplaces and execute changes needed in order to ensure continued safe work during pregnancy or breastfeeding. All assessments should be in accordance to national occupational health and safety acts, as well as maternity protection laws, which generally explain at which workplaces and under what conditions pregnant and breastfeeding women can work.
- Offer training courses on the implementation of maternity protection and risk assessments involving occupational physicians and the authorities responsible for occupational health and safety, with mandatory participation for chief physicians, supervisors, HR managers, works committee, and safety technology personnel.
- Develop a standard operating procedure (SOP) for a standardized approach after a pregnancy announcement involving management, a maternity protection officer, the company medical service, the safety technical service, occupational physicians, and the authorities responsible for occupational health and safety.
- Create an updated rotation plan for the period during and after pregnancy and maternity/ parental leave as part of such an SOP in the case of pregnancy during specialty training, with the aim of progressing in continuing education toward specialist status as quickly as possible.
- Use positive job lists from professional societies and associations aiding their implementation.
- Take joint precautions that simplify or continue to enable further work and specialty training in case of pregnancy symptoms (e.g., remote work, height-adjustable chairs and tables, recreation rooms).
- Develop a personnel concept that ensures an overlapping initial training of a pregnancy replacement.

17.2.9 Maternity Leave and Parental Leave

Many mother physicians have limited access to an adequate paid parental leave or fear risking career advancement, forcing them to return to work prematurely, face economic hardship, or gain financial dependence on their partner. In a profession characterized by constant innovations, parental leave also means an interruption of continuous learning. What to consider for maternity and parental leave in accordance with maternity and parental protection laws [10, 11, 32–34]:

- Provide comprehensive information on the possible financial burden of parental leave (e.g., implications on health insurance and pension fund) and strategies on how to address it.
- Implement comprehensive paid parental leave policies for both physician parents and medical students, if not already applicable due to maternity protection laws and parental leave laws.

- Expand the possibility of paid shared parental leave that can be taken jointly or additionally.
- Raise the assessment threshold for the entitlement to parental allowance to ensure that physicians have access to this social benefit, especially protecting mother physicians from financial dependence on their partner or the risk of reducing work hours beforehand in order to be entitled to parental allowance.
- Allow parents to return to work part-time during parental leave.
- Offer salary support during leave periods.
- Give the opportunity to maintain professional qualification during the parental leave period until re-entry, by enabling work, for example, as a sick or holiday replacement on an hourly basis (e.g., on-call duty).
- Give the opportunity to participate in departmental further education and training measures.
- Implement the same right for parent physicians on leave to participate in external training and qualification measures as physicians who are not on parental leave, as well as cover the costs.
- Establish comprehensive parental leave policies to encourage shared caregiving responsibilities without risking career advancement.
- Provide comprehensive parental leave policies to support bonding during crucial early development stages, explicitly including fathers/partners.

17.2.10 Returning from Leave and Lactation Period

It is important to ease the transition back to clinical practice after maternity/parental leave or adverse pregnancy outcomes (e.g., miscarriage) [10]. However, return from leave is usually made more difficult by inadequate or missing consultation from supervisors who are not taking into account the special needs of young mothers. How to help:

- Offer re-entry programs for physicians returning from extended family-related leaves [10], with documented conversations on tailored working conditions and pre-return engagement opportunities.
- Conduct a re-entry conversation addressing [33]
  - Wishes and interests with regard to re-entry
  - Possible date of re-entry
  - Part-time opportunities during and after parental leave
  - Agreement on binding working hours
  - Possible measures to obtain professional qualifications
  - Status and continuation of specialty training, doctorate, and/or habilitation in accordance with the regulations of the responsible medical association
  - Assessment of the possibilities from the supervisor's point of view
  - In the case of fixed-term employment relationships, the continuation of the employment relationship beyond the end of the fixed-term contract

Lack of time, space, and storage for pumping at work often forces mother physicians to choose between ending breastfeeding earlier than recommended or staying at home longer to enable breastfeeding for the desired duration with the acceptance of negative effects on professional advancement, pension fund, and other financial burden. How to support breastfeeding:

- Offer lactation support, including dedicated spaces and adequate time for breastfeeding or pumping, as well as providing appropriate storage facilities for expressed milk [10].
- Implement employer-provided childcare support, such as on-site crèches or parent–child offices.

17.2.11 Childcare and Children's Health

In an aging society, children become a demographic minority, just like the parents of underage children. It is necessary to actively advocate for their interests. Due to the increasing number of employed mothers, children today spend much more time in daycare and school than in the past. These widening and glaring gaps illustrate the enormously large and unpaid contribution (non-)employed mothers have been making in raising children and caring for relatives. So far, attempts have been made to replace their performance with quantity in care (e.g., all-day care). What has been lacking so far are high-quality educational offers combined with time and attention [35]. Parents justifiably demand that their children are not only kept safe, but also learn and receive attention while parents are committed to a functioning society and healthcare system with their work.

Working parents and employers can collaborate to create a supportive environment for children's healthy development, emphasizing the importance of strong attachments and supportive relationships. Here are key strategies:

Strategies for nationwide structural changes in childcare facilities and schools [35]:

- Equip them better.
- Compensate for the shortage of skilled workers by setting up multi-professional teams.
- Involve sports clubs, music schools, and other external education providers.
- Hire pensioners as paid freelancers (e.g., as reading mentors and for sports, music, or handicraft activities).
- Utilize highly educated unemployed such as recent college graduates, gap-year college students and pensioners to contribute to educating children in the classroom, at afterschool care facilities or at home (on-site or remotely)—analogous to the concept of the "Civilian College Corps" proposed by Claudia Goldin [36].
- Focus on the well-being of children with the importance of attachment figures.

Strategies for employers [9–11]:

- Foster an institutional culture that normalizes parenthood without straining colleagues, accepting that parental workforce can be diminished (e.g., due to chronic lack of sleep, absent days due to sickness or children's holidays), thereby increasing the workload on the colleagues present.
- Provide flexible work arrangements, remote work opportunities, IT systems for data exchange, and train more employees at the same skill level, when possible, to reconcile paid employment and family responsibilities.
- Implement employer-provided childcare support, such as on-site crèches or parent–child offices.
- Show empathy and provide flexibility.

Strategies for parents [3, 37, 38]:

- Prioritize quality time with children to foster secure attachments.
- Establish consistent routines and boundaries at home to provide stability and security for children.
- Exemplify positive behaviors and emotional regulation skills that children can emulate.
- Use government programs, if applicable, which support parental leave and allow parents to return to work part-time during parental leave.
- Participate in parent initiatives to create community-based childcare groups, fostering a supportive environment and allowing for greater parental involvement in children's care.
- Consider one parent starting work early and the other later, to ensure consistent parental presence and reduce reliance on external childcare, if needed.

17.2.12 Families with Diseases and Disabilities

Parents generally belong to an especially vulnerable group of employees as they have to care for their families, just like others caring for, for example, sick or elderly relatives. This comes with an increased need of security (e.g., financially). Parent physicians with disabilities or parent physicians having children with disabilities carry a special burden. The challenges they face may vary to a high extent in both groups. True participation, equality, and diversity can only exist if people with diseases and disabilities are considered equally valuable and worthy to be included. The following are key strategies for both parents and employers [39]:

Strategies for parents:

- Utilize flexible work arrangements, such as part-time options or adjustable hours, to accommodate both family responsibilities and health needs.
- Take advantage of the "severely handicapped pass" providing benefits such as special medical care, protection from dismissal, and support for childcare costs.
- Raise awareness among superiors and collegues on the condition, in order for them to understand individual needs and to be able to show solidarity.

Strategies for employers:

- Appreciate and utilize the skills of parents (with disabilities) such as problem-solving and empathetic patient management.
- Discuss openly, which professional commitment is feasible at which working hours.
- Make use of free consulting opportunities concerning inclusion offered by different national or local organizations.
- Introduce workplace accommodations and technical aids to implement necessary adjustments; many are eligible for government subsidies [40].
- Foster an institutional culture that exhibits acceptance for disability related needs, such as frequent absences, including doctors' appointments, or limited availability for extra hours.
- Show emotional support and understanding.

17.3 Radiology: A Good Specialty Choice for Parents?

In times of an increasing skilled worker shortage, radiology can position itself as a family-friendly specialty that offers both career satisfaction and the ability to prioritize family life. The changes needed for this transformation have the potential to attract many physicians regardless of their private situation. The following provides key strategies for [8, 18, 41]:

Addressing workflow and working conditions:

- Implement flexible work arrangements, including part-time options, predictable schedules with adjustable hours and remote work opportunities (e.g., teleradiology, teaching, organizational tasks, research). This eases childcare planning, allowing for a better compatibility of paid employment and family life and thus increasing overall well-being.
- Utilize the opportunity to hire retired specialists as freelancers to take over shifts in the afternoon and evening for regular workload, and supervise/teach physicians in specialty training.
- Implement scheduling systems that allow radiologists to customize their workload and income goals, providing control over their professional and personal lives.
- Implement integrated Radiology Information System (RIS) and Picture Archiving and Communication System (PACS) solutions to streamline workflows and improve efficiency.
- Integrate AI education into medical education and specialty training to alleviate concerns about its impact on the field of radiology, as well as highlight how AI can enhance rather than replace the radiologist's role.
- Foster the future potential for practice-based work, strengthening the medical profession in times of rising private-equity financial investors in the healthcare sector.

Addressing parents and parents-to-be:

- Utilize the potential and implement changes needed for a functioning compatibility of paid employment and family life (including both unpaid care work and quality time) in radiology to attract more women to the field.
- Offer mentorship programs and support networks for radiologists with families, helping them navigate career advancement while managing family responsibilities.
- Implement comprehensive paid parental leave policies to support new parents in their career and family life for those not applicable to maternity protection laws and parental leave laws.
- Provide lactation facilities and appropriate time for breastfeeding mothers, ensuring that they can continue their professional duties while meeting their own and their children's needs.

Addressing medical students:

- Improve the medical curriculum and implement mentorship to enhance interest in radiology among medical students.
- Address concerns about limited patient interaction by providing more hands-on experiences to highlight radiology's impact on patient care (e.g., interventional radiology, angiography).
- Address concerns about limited interaction with co-workers in radiology by showcasing the field's interdisciplinary nature (e.g., tumor boards).

17.4 Discussion

Supporting Parent Physicians in Medicine

Improving work integration and career support for parent physicians, particularly mother physicians, who are especially affected by work–life (im-)balance issues is pivotal for training and retaining skilled professionals, promoting gender equity, and fostering holistic lifestyles in medicine [18]. Parenthood represents a fundamental societal task that benefits everyone. Yet, the medical profession often places undue pressure on mothers, creating unrealistic expectations to excel simultaneously in career, caregiving, and personal well-being. This environment can be demoralizing, leading many women to scale back or leave medicine entirely [3, 4, 25], creating an outcome that is unsustainable in the face of demographic challenges and skilled worker shortages.

A significant cultural shift is necessary to move from downplaying or concealing parental responsibilities to celebrating them as dual achievements. Parenthood equips individuals with valuable skills, such as multitasking, time management, and emotional intelligence, which can then enhance their professional performance. However, the prevailing "all-or-nothing" mentality—that only those working full-time can succeed as physicians—needs to be replaced with flexible approaches that accommodate both varied career trajectories and private choices [16, 28]. Empowering parent physicians to choose their paths without judgment or structural disadvantage is essential.

Key Challenges and Strategies

1. *Unrealistic expectations and pressure*:

   Mothers face pressure to "do it all," leading to guilt or inadequacy when striving to reconcile their family and career. Medicine must redefine success by moving away from a culture of "greedy work" that often forces women to choose between career advancement and family responsibilities. Instead, it must perpetuate inequality in the workplace toward a family-friendly environment that allows for part-time work, flexible hours, remote work, and personalized career pacing [9]. Institutions should normalize and support diverse employment arrangements, ensuring that physicians who prioritize family responsibilities can still undergo specialty training and access specialty status, leadership roles, and professional advancement.
2. *Cultural and institutional change* [17, 31]:

   A persistent bias implies that women should have foregone medical careers if they wanted children. This harmful narrative must be replaced by affirmations that parenting and medicine can coexist. Medical education and specialty training programs should emphasize this compatibility, fostering supportive cultures from the outset. Supportive work environments emphasize collegiality, recognition, and open dialogue.
3. *Equity and inclusion*:

   Addressing systemic inequalities and discrimination requires tailored support for parents, especially mother physicians, including those with disabilities. Transparent policies on specialty training, research programs, career options, maternal/parental leave, and retirement contributions among others must be integrated into institutional frameworks.
4. *Work infrastructure*:

   Many medical institutions lack the sufficient (infra-)structural requirements for the continued employment of women physicians subject to maternity protection laws, such as on-site childcare, and resources for flexible part-time employment. Addressing these gaps requires [10, 12]:

   - Workplace adaptation: Having an SOP that includes a positive interpretation of maternity protection laws, is under implementation of legal requirements for pregnancies, and is adequately protecting both mother and child from physical or psychological impairments.
   - Equitable parental leave: Providing adequate pregnancy and maternity/parental leave policies (e.g., adapted rotation plans before/after leave, supporting both parents, encouraging shared caregiving responsibilities without risking career advancement), easing the transition back to clinical practice after leave and in cases of, for example, miscarriage.

- Enhanced childcare options: Offering breastfeeding places, on-site childcare facilities, emergency childcare solutions, or subsidies for external services.
- Flexible scheduling: Leveraging telemedicine and technology to enable remote work and adjustable work hours, as well as shared (top-)job models.

5. *Supporting career transitions* [8, 13, 15]:
   Many physicians fear disclosing their desire to have children due to potential career repercussions. Institutions should create safe environments where parenting and everything involved are viewed positively. Providing mentoring programs and networking opportunities can help physicians navigate transitions, ensuring continuity in career development.
6. *Specialty choice*:
   The specialties adopting these measures enhance their appeal and strengthen their workforce for future challenges. Radiology offers great potential to play a leading role in supporting both family and career.
7. *Specialty training* [5, 8, 10, 12, 19–24]:
   Positive interpretation of maternity protection laws and customized flexible rotation plans facilitate qualifications toward specialist status despite pregnancy, maternal/paternal leave, and parental responsibilities after reentry.

Long-Term Benefits

Comprehensive support for parent physicians leads to multiple benefits [8, 9, 12, 13, 42–44]:

- Enhanced job satisfaction and motivation, particularly in supportive environments.
- Retention of talented professionals, ensuring continuity of care and expertise
- Improved patient outcomes through consistent diverse and inclusive healthcare teams
- Contribution to closing the Gender Pay Gap, Gender Lifetime Earnings Gap, and Gender Pension Gap

In conclusion, creating parent-friendly structures in medicine requires a multifaceted approach that combines policy reform, cultural change, and institutional commitment. By embracing flexibility and inclusivity, medical institutions can ensure that physicians thrive as professionals and parents, ultimately strengthening the entire healthcare system. These reforms are essential for addressing equity, participation, and workforce shortages while maintaining excellence in patient care and research amidst evolving healthcare demands.

Medical practice is guided by a fundamental ethical understanding, as reflected in the Geneva Pledge, which emphasizes the importance of self-care and well-being for physicians to provide optimal patient care, including the right to self-determination for pregnant doctors, ultimately contributing to professional satisfaction and a supportive work environment [5, 12, 45].

Radiology, characterized by its unique intersection of advanced imaging technology, patient-focused diagnostics and intervention, as well as innovative research in an interdisciplinary setting, provides an ideal environment for enacting reforms that support parent physicians and those wishing to become parents. By leveraging flexible work structures, remote work opportunities, and predictable scheduling, the specialty can lead in creating family-friendly policies that attract and retain diverse talent [8].

Research on physician parents and medical students with children remains limited. More comprehensive studies are needed to

- Evaluate the effectiveness of existing support policies
- Understand the long-term career impacts of parenting in medicine
- Develop evidence-based interventions to support physician-parents

17.5 Conclusion

Family-friendly medical institutions take into account the special features associated with them, such as responding to pregnancy, breastfeeding, and parenthood with a supportive work environment. Acknowledging and utilizing the professional commitment feasible during different stages of pregnancy and parenthood is the key to leverage workforce potential in times of demographic change and skilled worker shortages. Providing both a supportive infrastructure and institutional culture by implementing the structural changes listed above will contribute to the empowerment of many skilled workers to participate in the job market, conducing to a successful healthcare system.

The employers getting through the upcoming challenges most sustainably will be those willing to create a truly family-friendly environment that provides flexible career paths that support parents with their everyday life of having a career and family. Professional societies and associations adapting an "employer branding" as such with comprehensive modern conditions for both work and specialty training will attract future generations of physicians and manage to build up and retain skilled professionals for their specialties. Radiology has great potential to take a leading role.

The motto is: enable participation according to all possibilities, but respect and support the personal decisions of the individual parents. Having children is one of the most personal circumstances of all. Parents want to spend as much time with their children as possible, being there to raise and accompany them as they grow up. This is never a decision against work, but rather for their offspring. A supportive work environment, modern infrastructure, and high-quality childcare will ease parents on their individual journey of the compatibility and combining of family and career.

Literature

1. de Vries A(E-H), Shamseer L, Bourgeault I, Grunfeld E, Moore A, Peer N, Straus SE, Tricco AC. Will COVID-19 result in a giant step backwards for women in academic science? J Clin Epidemiol. 2021;134:160–6. https://doi.org/10.1016/j.jclinepi.2021.03.004.
2. Davis PB, Meagher EA, Pomeroy C, Lowe WL, Rubenstein AH, Wu JY, Curtis AB, Jackson RD. The impact of COVID-19 on the careers of women in academic sciences, engineering, and medicine // Pandemic-related barriers to the success of women in research: a framework for action. Nat Med. 2021/2022;28(3):436–8. https://doi.org/10.1038/s41591-022-01692-8.
3. Juengst SB, Royston A, Huang I, Wright B. Family leave and return-to-work experiences of physician mothers. JAMA Netw Open. 2019;2(10):e1913054. https://doi.org/10.1001/jamanetworkopen.2019.13054.
4. Casilla-Lennon M, Hanchuk S, Zheng S, Kim DD, Press B, Nguyen JV, Grimshaw A, Leapman MS, Cavallo JA. Pregnancy in physicians: a scoping review. Am J Surg. 2022;223(1):36–46. https://doi.org/10.1016/j.amjsurg.2021.07.011.
5. Bündnis Junge Ärztinnen und Ärzte, AG Junge Gastroenterologie der DGVS, Young DGN. Positionspapier zur ärztlichen Weiterbildung anlässlich der Krankenhausreform - Die Weiterbildung muss mitgedacht werden -: ein gemeinsames Positionspapier des Bündnis Junge Ärztinnen und Ärzte und der AG Junge Gastroenterologie der DGVS sowie der Young DGN [Internet]; 2023 [cited 2025 Feb 27]. p. 11. Available from: https://www.forum-junge-radiologie.de/themes/free/jurad/downloads/BJA-Positionspapier-aerztliche-Weiterbildung-anlaesslich-Krankenhausreform-Stand-2024-01-10.pdf.
6. Chesak SS, Yngve KC, Taylor JM, Voth ER, Bhagra A. Challenges and solutions for physician mothers: a critical review of the literature. Mayo Clin Proc. 2021;96(6):1578–91. https://doi.org/10.1016/j.mayocp.2020.10.008.
7. Di Bartolo B, Torres IL. Motherhood penalty and the gender gap in STEM and medicine. Eur Heart J. 2024;45(31):2800–2. https://doi.org/10.1093/eurheartj/ehae262.
8. See E, Herold C, Bamberg F, Ljimani A. Vereinbarkeit von Schwangerschaft, Elternschaft, Ärztlicher Weiterbildung und Karriere in der Radiologie [Reconciling pregnancy, parenthood, medical training and a career in radiology]. Radiologie (Heidelb). 2024;64(12):956–9. https://doi.org/10.1007/s00117-024-01379-w.
9. Goldin CD. Career & family: women's century-long journey toward equity, vol. 1. Princeton: Princeton university press; 2021. p. XII–325.
10. Rangel EL. Work-life integration in medicine: a movement, not a mandate. JAMA Netw Open. 2023;6(1):e2250957. https://doi.org/10.1001/jamanetworkopen.2022.50957.
11. Quigley L. Helping working parents avoid burnout: a guide for employers [Internet]. HRD Connect; 2024 [cited 2025 Jan 28]. Available from: https://www.hrdconnect.com/2024/10/09/helping-working-parents-avoid-burnout-a-guide-for-employers/.
12. Nordrhein Ä, Workshop Mutterschutz. Arbeiten in der Schwangerschaft (und Stillzeit) - Forderungen zur Verbesserung der Lage von Ärztinnen. Positionspapier des Workshop Mutterschutz [Internet]; 2023 [cited 2025 Feb 27]. p. 9. Available from: https://www.aekno.de/fileadmin/user_upload/aekno/downloads/2024/positionspapier-mutterschutz-2024-12.pdf.
13. Capron RA. The role that mentors play in women's work life balance [Internet]. Pepperdine University; 2014 [cited 2025 Feb 27]. p. 140. Available from: https://digitalcommons.pepperdine.edu/etd/491.
14. Darves B. Physician mentorship: why it's important, and how to find and sustain relationships [Internet]; 2018 [cited 2025 Feb 27]. Available from: https://resources.nejmcareercenter.org/article/physician-mentorship-why-its-important-and-how-to-find-and-sustain-relationships/.
15. Berg S. Supporting physician mothers on their journey [Internet]. American Medical Association; 2019 [cited 2025 Jan 28]. Available from: https://www.ama-assn.org/delivering-care/health-equity/supporting-physician-mothers-their-journey.
16. Olazagasti C, Florez N. Work-life balance vs. work-life integration: a young physician mother's journey. The Oncologist. 2022;27(11):991–2. https://doi.org/10.1093/oncolo/oyac175.

17. Dason ES, Maxim M, Gesink D, Yee M, Chan C, Baxter NN, Shapiro H, Simpson AN. Medical students' perspectives on family planning and impact on specialty choice. JAMA Surg. 2024;159(2):170–8. https://doi.org/10.1001/jamasurg.2023.6392.
18. Rich A, Viney R, Needleman S, Griffin A, Woolf K. 'You can't be a person and a doctor': the work-life balance of doctors in training-a qualitative study. BMJ Open. 2016;6(12):e013897. https://doi.org/10.1136/bmjopen-2016-013897.
19. Arnold H. Bündnis JUNGE ÄRZTE: Positionspapier: Vereinbarkeit von Familie und Karriere - wo bleibt der Wandel in den Köpfen? [Bündnis JUNGE ÄRZTE: position paper: Compatibility of family and career - where is the change in minds?]. Der Urologe. Ausg. A. 2016;55(6):821–2. https://doi.org/10.1007/s00120-016-0111-8.
20. Caperelli Gergel MC, Terry DL. Giving 200%: workplace flexibility and provider distress among female physicians. J Healthc Leadersh. 2022;14:83–9. https://doi.org/10.2147/JHL.S359389.
21. Fortmann C, Johna S, Groß C, Niethard M, Puhahn-Schmeiser B. Obstacles during training of pregnant doctors in Germany before and after COVID-19: Is there a need for change? Innov Surg Sci. 2024; https://doi.org/10.1515/iss-2024-0021.
22. Oechtering TH, Panagiotopoulos N, Völker M, Lohwasser S, Ellmann S, Molwitz I, et al. Arbeits- und Weiterbildungsbedingungen in der Facharztweiterbildung Radiologie—Ergebnisse einer bundesweiten Weiterbildungsumfrage durch das Forum Junge Radiologie in der Deutschen Röntgengesellschaft. Rofo. 2020;192(5):458–70. https://doi.org/10.1055/a-1047-1075.
23. See E, Kerner DS, Luther A, Richardt D, Herrmann H, Groß C, Witt V, Martini I, Lux H, Trittmacher S, Polkowski C. Rahmenbedingungen zur Verbesserung der Vereinbarkeit von ärztlicher Erwerbstätigkeit und Sorgearbeit gesetzlich verankern [Internet]. Mainz: 128. Deutscher Ärztetag; 2024 [cited 2025 Feb 27]. p. 1. Available from: https://128daet.baek.de/data/media/BIc90.pdf.
24. See E, Kerner DS, Richardt D, Groß C, Martini I, Luther A, Lux H, Fach WA, Trittmacher S, Polkowski C. Rahmenbedingungen zum Erhalt der Arbeitskraft und zur Fortführung der ärztlichen Weiterbildung in Schwangerschaft, Stillzeit, Elternschaft und anderer Sorgearbeit in der Familie gesetzlich verankern [Internet]: 128. Deutscher Ärztetag; 2024 [cited 2025 Feb 27]. p. 2. Available from: https://128daet.baek.de/data/media/BIIId04.pdf.
25. Buddeberg-Fischer B, Stamm M, Buddeberg C, Bauer G, Hämmig O, Knecht M, Klaghofer R. The impact of gender and parenthood on physicians' careers - professional and personal situation seven years after graduation. BMC Health Serv Res. 2010:1040. https://doi.org/10.1186/1472-6963-10-40.
26. Simpson AN, Cusimano MC, Baxter NN. The inconvenience of motherhood during a medical career. CMAJ. 2021;193(37):E1465–6. https://doi.org/10.1503/cmaj.211255.
27. Morgan HK, Singer K, Fitzgerald JT, Brower KJ, Spencley BM, Owens LE, Burrows HL. Perceptions of parenting challenges and career progression among physician faculty at an Academic Hospital. JAMA Netw Open. 2020;3(12):e2029076. https://doi.org/10.1001/jamanetworkopen.2020.29076.
28. Deutsche Forschungsgemeinschaft. More flexible career paths for clinician scientists: DFG Senate Commission has developed proposals concerning career prospects for clinician scientists/The long-term aim is to boost university medicine [Internet]; 2024 [cited 2025 Feb 27]. Available from: https://www.dfg.de/en/service/press/press-releases/2024/press-release-no-34.
29. Malhotra A, Futela D, Joshi R, Payabvash S, White B, Seidenwurm D, Gandhi D, Duszak R. Recent trends in academic versus nonacademic radiologist compensation and clinical productivity. J Am Coll Radiol: JACR. 2024;S1546-1440(24):00910–4. https://doi.org/10.1016/j.jacr.2024.10.020.
30. Prokosch-Willing V, Hos D, Joachim SC. Forschung in der Weiterbildung. Ophthalmologe. 2017;114(10):901–5. https://doi.org/10.1007/s00347-017-0566-z.
31. Dason ES, Kapsack A, Baxter NN, Gesink D, Shapiro H, Simpson AN. Resident and fellow perspectives on family planning and building during training. JAMA Netw Open. 2024;7(8):e2429345. https://doi.org/10.1001/jamanetworkopen.2024.29345.

32. Bundesministerium für Familie, Senioren, Frauen und Jugend. Gesetz zum Elterngeld und zur Elternzeit (Bundeselterngeld- und Elternzeitgesetz - BEEG); 2006 [cited 2025 Jan 29]. Available from: https://www.gesetze-im-internet.de/beeg/BJNR274810006.html.
33. Bund M, Hessen L. Tarifvertrag für die Ärztinnen und Ärzte an den hessischen Universitätskliniken (TV-Ärzte Hessen) vom 30. November 2006: in der Fassung des Änderungstarifvertrages Nr. 11 vom 24. Mai 2024 [Internet] [cited 2025 Feb 27]. p. 32. Available from: https://www.marburger-bund.de/sites/default/files/tarifvertraege/2024-12/TV-%C3%84rzte%20Hessen%20Unikliniken.pdf.
34. European Union. DIRECTIVE (EU) 2019/1158 OF THE EUROPEAN PARLIAMENT AND OF THE COUNCIL - of 20 June 2019 - on work-life balance for parents and carers and repealing Council Directive 2010/18/EU [Internet] [cited 2025 Feb 27]; p. 15. Available from: https://eur-lex.europa.eu/legal-content/EN/TXT/PDF/?uri=CELEX:32019L1158.
35. Otto J, Schoener J. Kinderbetreuung- "Der Staat kann nicht die Mütter ersetzen" | ZEIT ONLINE: Zeit; 2025 [cited 2025 Jan 29]. Available from: URL: https://www.zeit.de/2025/03/kinderbetreuung-muetter-kindergarten-schule-demografischer-wandel.
36. Goldin C. The 2020 Martin S. Feldstein Lecture - Journey across a Century of Women [Internet]. NBER Reporter; 2020 [cited 2025 Jan 21]. p. 36. Available from: https://live-nber.pantheonsite.io/sites/default/files/2020-10/reporter-2020-03.pdf.
37. Myers R. Balancing work and family: tips for working parents [Internet]. Child Development Institute. 2024 [updated 2025 Feb 27]. Available from: https://childdevelopmentinfo.com/parenting/balancing-work-and-family-tips-for-working-parents/.
38. Merrill S, Sheehan J. Building positive learning environments for young children starts with you [Internet]. U.S. Department of Health & Human Services; 2018 [cited 2025 Feb 27]. Available from: https://headstart.gov/blog/building-positivc-learning-environments-young-children-starts-you.
39. Katharina Ronstedt, interviewed on 27.01.2025 as speaker of the network Diversity@DRG and co-founder of its focus group YesWeCanToo/disability@DRG.
40. Federal Anti-Discrimination Agency. Guide to the general equal treatment act: explanations and examples. Federal Anti-Discrimination Agency; 2019. [cited 2025 Feb 27] Available from: URL: https://www.antidiskriminierungsstelle.de/SharedDocs/downloads/EN/publikationen/agg_wegweiser_engl_guide_to_the_general_equal_treatment_act.pdf?__blob=publicationFile#:~:text=The%20objective%20of%20the%20General,%2C%20age%2C%20or%20sexual%20orientation.&text=Employers%20have%20legally%20mandated%20organisational%20obligations.
41. Christoffel I, Zhong J, Ho R, Gourtsoyianni S, Oleaga L, Catalano C, Becker M, Goh V. Attracting the next generation of radiologists: a statement by the European Society of Radiology (ESR) // Attracting the next generation of radiologists: a statement by the European Society of Radiology (ESR). Insights Imaging. 2022;13(1):84. https://doi.org/10.1186/s13244-022-01221-8.
42. Jones LK, Jennings BM, Higgins MK, de Waal FBM. Ethological observations of social behavior in the operating room. Proc Natl Acad Sci U S A. 2018;115(29):7575–80. https://doi.org/10.1073/pnas.1716883115.
43. Miyawaki A, Jena AB, Rotenstein LS, Tsugawa Y. Comparison of hospital mortality and readmission rates by physician and patient sex. Ann Intern Med. 2024;177(5):598–608. https://doi.org/10.7326/M23-3163.
44. Wallis CJD, Jerath A, Coburn N, et al. Association of surgeon-patient sex concordance with postoperative outcomes. JAMA Surg. 2022;157(2):146–56. https://doi.org/10.1001/jamasurg.2021.6339.
45. The World Medical Association. WMA declaration of Geneva; 2017 [cited 2025 Feb 27]. Available from: https://www.wma.net/policies-post/wma-declaration-of-geneva/.

18 Inclusion Extended to People with Disability

Katharina Ronstedt

18.1 Level of "Inclusion" in the German General Labor Market

Legally speaking, the situation for people with disabilities is quite favorable. Germany not only signed the United Nations Convention on the Rights of Persons with Disabilities (UNCRPD) in March 2007 and ratified it in New York [1] in February 2009, but also implemented it in the Federal Participation Law. One of the aims of this law is to promote the participation of people with disabilities [2]. To this end, it offers various benefits for employers and employees alike. Other laws that promote the same objective are the Law on Equal Opportunities for Persons with Disabilities, which was implied between 2017 and 2023 and focuses on public participation and self-advocacy, and the General Equal Treatment Act [3], (August 2006) mainly concerns protection in various aspects of the labor market. The Act to Promote an Inclusive Labor Market (January 2024) saw the introduction of much stricter financial penalties for employers with 20 or more employees failing to meet the 5% quota for the hiring of severely (degree of disability at least 50) disabled individuals.

While it might be assumed that this is a reasonable level of protection, analyses of current employment levels indicate the ineffectiveness of these measures: Only 4.44% of all jobs are filled by people with severe disabilities, which in other words means that there is a gap of 73,000 jobs to be filled by people with disabilities in order to reach the legal target of 5.0%. Despite all efforts, the increase in employment of disabled people has not exceeded the improvement in the general labor market in recent years [4].

K. Ronstedt (✉)
Department of Pediatric Radiology, Kassel Hospital GmbH, Kassel, Germany
e-mail: Katharina.Ronstedt@gnh.net

S. Keller-Yamamura, J. Yamamura (eds.), *Inclusive Radiology: Fostering Diversity and Equity in Academic and non-Academic Settings*,
https://doi.org/10.1007/978-3-032-05705-1_18

Companies are assessed on the basis of their overall employment rate, without differentiating according to wages or training requirements. This masks the even more pronounced under-representation of highly qualified workers.

The cause of this can be found even earlier in life: Education is regulated at the level of the Länder, whereas integration law is a federal matter, which means that the socio-legal protection described above does not apply during education, and the definition of "special needs" can even lead to partial exclusion of impaired pupils from regular schools or to compulsory attendance at schools for the disabled. This leads to an even higher level of insecurity and discrimination during education and training than later in life [5].

In particular, young people who aspire to a career in the high-wage segment, or simply an academic degree, are more vulnerable to the inconsistency of regulations and may not be able to perform according to their abilities due to discrimination or an unwillingness to meet their needs [2].

In the United States, the proportion of medical school graduates who have a relevant physical impairment is less than 0.5% [6]. This data is from 2016, but there is little hope that these numbers have increased significantly. Nor is there any evidence that impaired individuals in Germany are much better off, as there are no better regulations in higher education for them.

18.2 Inclusion of People with Disability in Healthcare: qui bono?

Though no statistics are available concerning the number of professionals in medicine suffering severe impairment, the absolute number of individuals who are impaired since childhood, as well as those who have gained impairment over the course of their lives, shall be considered high enough to consider this group as an underrecognized treasure of talents.

Individuals living with disabilities who have successfully completed medical or paramedical studies contribute unique skills and perspectives to the healthcare sector. Their high level of intrinsic motivation and well-developed problem-solving abilities make them valuable members of an inclusive team.

There is quite some data indicating that people with disabilities experience high levels of healthcare inequities [6], which result in poorer health outcomes unrelated to their underlying disability [7]. One might hypothesize that an institution that fails to allocate enabling resources to the needs of employees is unlikely to be able to meet the special needs of patients either. Individuals with experiential knowledge of addressing challenges posed by physical conditions may serve as valuable resources in facilitating access to this demographic of patients [8].

An inclusive work environment is particularly appealing to young professionals. An inclusive work environment not only fosters diversity, but also provides a space where individuals can thrive without the pressure to fully conform. Research indicates that diversity and inclusion in healthcare are conducive to innovation as different perspectives converge and novel approaches emerge [9].

Furthermore, individuals living with impairments frequently have experienced discrimination and are therefore often loyal employees who truly appreciate being treated fairly. Their commitment and dedication contribute to team stability and can strengthen staff retention [10].

Consequently, the promotion of inclusion for disabled healthcare professionals is not merely an ethical imperative, but also a strategically advantageous approach for the healthcare sector.

18.3 Diversity Without Inclusion?

In the context of the workplace, "diversity" is by definition no more than the quantitative description of a certain status. It simply describes the presence and extent of differences in a group. This includes gender, ethnicity, age, sexual orientation, or whatever other characteristic is deemed worthy of representation [11].

Inclusion, on the other hand, is a more qualitative term and, if you like, a call to action. It focuses on the experiences of people with different dimensions of diversity in a given environment [12].

Unlike in academic and management research, the two terms are often confused in current public debate, which leads to the misunderstanding that allowing individuals with disabilities to become part of a team is named "inclusion," while doing the same with a person of color is standing up for diversity [13].

While the value of diversifying the medical workforce in terms of gender and race is widely accepted [14, 12] the need to extend the concept to people with disabilities is not [14]. Unfortunately, this also applies to radiology [15]. Therefore, we will focus on the inclusion of people with disabilities and discuss enablers and barriers to achieving a higher level of diversity in radiology.

18.4 "Them People" Share Many Similarities, While Some Aspects Differ

In her capacity as spokesperson for the DRG's diversity network, the author possesses a comprehensive understanding of the endeavors and challenges faced by the various focus groups. In addition to the group that is committed to inclusion of people with disability "yes-we-can-too," whose experiences we will discuss below, the group that caters to people with a history of migration in radiology and the group of women in radiology are particularly active.

It is noteworthy that a considerable proportion of the challenges faced by individuals from diverse backgrounds are interconnected.

1. The majority have encountered a professional context that intermittently focuses on one aspect of their overall personality, rather than the entirety of their multifaceted identities.

1.1. The accentuation of a single characteristic is frequently linked to a diminution in professional reliability and competence. This attribution is frequently made by colleagues and managers who have limited or no personal experience in dealing with this characteristic, both personally and professionally. This evaluation is frequently adopted by others within the team or tacitly endorsed.
2. The actual difficulty in everyday working life that a team experiences due to a certain characteristic of an employee is not seen in relation to the benefit that the team member brings to the group.
2.2. The impairment is often seen as a personal fault or failure of the individual, the compensation for which can only be realized by the person concerned.
3. The groups in the diversity network are regarded as safe spaces where mutual understanding is facilitated. These groups facilitate open dialogue and problem-solving, encouraging a shift from individual needs to a more systematic approach.
4. It is evident that a number of the projects undertaken by the various groups have garnered recognition within the radiology community. This recognition has led to an increase in the reputation of the respective representatives as experts in various aspects of diversity. Consequently, these groups have become recognized as sources of consultation for those seeking to embrace more progressive approaches.

Although only a minority of those calling for a more diverse radiology workforce are physically disabled, they share all of the above experiences.

Although inclusion is always a challenge for an entire organization or department, and its needs extend to all people who were not originally thought of as part of the establishment, each marginalized group, including people with disabilities, has specific challenges.

The following are particularly serious (*examples from the Diversity Network's consultancy work are in italics*):

1. Physical disability is stigmatized. The assumption that a team member is not contributing fully because of their impairment is not only widespread, but is often not reflected in the extent of real or only assumed underperformance. Furthermore, it is assumed that there is no way to improve performance by adjusting the circumstances [16].

   A young radiology specialist in a substantial secondary care facility experiences ambulation difficulties. Notwithstanding this, he has worked night shifts for a period exceeding 4 years at the hospital where he aspires to advance his professional career. It is noteworthy that there has been no recorded instance of patient safety being compromised by this individual's condition, nor has his absence from work been more prolonged than that of his colleagues. When he inquired about a promotion, he was informed that his performance was not on par with that of his colleagues and that he should wait a few more years before making another request. Subsequently, upon the presentation of quantitative evidence that sought to substantiate his claim of equitable performance, he was informed that not all pertinent elements were quantifiable.

2. It is often assumed that the individual is to blame for the fact that other colleagues have to work more because of them and that they therefore contribute to overloading their "healthy" colleagues. These insinuations are usually made regardless of whether there were candidates who could have performed better in the position [17].
3. People with nonobvious disabilities often try to hide them in order to avoid the negative attributions associated with disability. This hiding takes up a lot of energy that could be better spent learning and performing in the job itself [17, 18].

   A medical doctor in the early stages of her career, who had recently qualified and was interested in pursuing a specialty in radiology, was offered a position at a local hospital where there were three vacant positions for residents. Due to her juvenile diabetes, she was advised to refrain from night shifts and disclose her condition, including the potential need for assistance. However, she was counseled by a diabetic colleague from a different medical discipline, who advised her to conceal her condition and accept a less favorable glycemic control, as he found it difficult to cope with the microaggressions he was experiencing as a result of his exemption from night work. The young colleague expressed a predominant fear of being blamed for underperformance and consequently opted to disclose her condition while reassuring her superiors of her ability to provide a 24-hour on-call service. However, within a period of less than 6 months, she experienced a major hypoglycemia during a night shift, necessitating treatment in the emergency room. It was only then that she dared to speak up and explain how difficult it was to maintain stable blood glucose levels while working shifts. Subsequently, she overheard fellow residents voicing their discontent regarding her employment, while conveniently overlooking the fact that there were still vacancies in the department.
4. Stigma is often much stronger in the professional context than at university or school, which can lead to a loss of self-esteem. This emotional distress can affect an individual's mental well-being to such an extent that their level of performance is significantly impaired [19].
5. As there are very few obviously physically disabled professionals in a hospital, the impairment is often seen as the most outstanding characteristic of a member of staff. As a result, many feel reduced to this one characteristic, while their other qualities are ignored [20].

   A radiology attending who has experienced hearing impairment since childhood has relocated to a new workplace and wishes to ensure that his previous employment and incapacitation for several months remain undisclosed. As rumors began to circulate, he felt compelled to address the situation, and so he sought consultation with the helpline. In his previous professional role, he was frequently referred to as the "deaf man" or the "deaf radiologist." The subject is notably tall, wears horn-rimmed glasses, has a distinctive face, loves to travel, and is a good cook, but nothing distinguishes him as much as his hearing aids and his need to lip-read. His hearing impairment required heightened concentration and focus during medical rounds and discussions. On occasion, he found it necessary to request repetition of what had been said. Consequently, these two factors together began to cause him to disidentify as an integral part of his team. As time passed, he began to feel increasingly excluded and rumored to be the source of discreet whispers and gossip. This emotional burden ultimately led to dysthymia, and, subsequently, a severe depression. After a period of treatment, he regained the strength to continue working in radiology, but saw no way to return to the department.

He found some solace in the fact that many individuals with impairment have had similar experiences and that, to the best of our knowledge, no one has yet found the perfect way to manage this.

6. There is a notable lack of role models [21].

   The authors' thesis counselor suffers from the same condition as the author herself. Due to the fact that the impairment is not visible, it was possible for him to conceal it during his education. During her own time as a medical student working in his department, she gained valuable insights into effective strategies for managing disabilities. Through his own actions, he demonstrated that work and cooperative tasks can be more efficiently and productively executed when individual requirements are taken into account. This principle transcends disability, encompassing language barriers, pregnancy, and familial responsibilities. The creation of an atmosphere in which individuals can address their needs and discuss options openly is a core responsibility of the head of department. He never expressed any doubt that someone with special needs might not be fit for running a department, so she inhaled that assumption as a truth before she even started residency. The majority of physically impaired doctors do not have the luxury of being able to entertain the notion that pursuing professional ambitions is a realistic prospect for them, and instead find themselves preoccupied with the question of how such ambitions might be realized.

18.5 Impairment Versus Disability

Lisa, a junior doctor in her third year of further training in radiology, aspires to undertake radiology demonstrations autonomously. She has a particular interest in neuroradiology and is therefore initially asked to demonstrate in the neurology department. Noteworthy is that Liz suffers from dysarthria. This condition has had minimal impact on her professional performance thus far, as she is highly proficient in utilizing the dictation system, which enables her to produce reports with an only modest increase in time. The repetition of syllables is the impairment, while the additional time required to produce findings is the disability. In this particular instance, the impact of the impairment is relatively manageable.

Conversely, in circumstances involving comprehensive examinations of poly trauma patients in the ER, the impact on her speech condition is much more pronounced. Accordingly, she has reached a consensus with her clinical colleagues on the utilization of concise expressions, which convey the essential information without necessitating the formation of complex words or sentences. This approach, therefore, has led to a substantial reduction in the impact of her disability, arising from the aforementioned impairment and from the situation itself.

Her first interdisciplinary round takes place in the midst of colleagues who are not very understanding and who keep interrupting her or are obviously annoyed by her stuttering. She is unable to present her findings in a coherent manner due to the frequent disruptions she experiences. As her stress levels increase, she is unable to respond adequately to inquiries. The following day, the head neurologist approached Lisa's consultant and asked her to hand over the round to another colleague as the findings presentation was mediocre and the time taken was too long. The colleague taking over already has several scheduled demonstrations and is experiencing elevated levels of stress. He expresses feelings of unfairness regarding the additional workload.

The degree of impairment does not necessarily translate into the extent of disability. The American Medical Association offers a more distinct approach and provides the following definition:

Impairment—"any marked loss or deviation in physiological function, psychological function, or anatomical structure of the body …" [22]·

Disability—"the impact of impairment on a person's ability to meet the demands of his or her life." [22]

The nature of both conditions can be temporary or permanent, worsening or improving over time. Of paramount importance is that these changes do not invariably occur concurrently [23]. The extent of the impairment is only discernible in the individual concerned and can, if at all, be influenced by treating the condition. Conversely, the extent of the disability is contingent on the respective social circumstances, in this case professional, and can be influenced by the affected individual and stakeholders in the environment [24].

Nevertheless, particularly within the German language, these terms are often employed indistinguishably. As language shapes perception, these inaccuracies reinforce the tendency to place much of the burden of impairment in a professional setting on the individual. Consequently, those responsible often neglect to consider modifications to the working environment, thereby hindering team members from fulfilling their core professional duties.

18.6 You Are the One Who Is Impaired? It Is Up to You to Press for Change

There is some positive news to report: The scarcity of skilled labor is advantageous for us [25], the laws mentioned above are increasingly being enforced in the healthcare sector and the call for more diversity allows people with disabilities to draw attention to shared interests, and more and more healthcare professionals with disabilities are being appointed to decision-making positions.

However, there is still much to be done. While advocates of inclusion hail from a diverse array of backgrounds, individuals with impairments remain significantly underrepresented. This is a challenge that can only be confronted by those with disabilities themselves.

The subsequent recommendations, while not backed by scientific research, are derived from peer counseling, shared experiences and feedback from different stakeholders.

18.7 During the Application Phase

If an applicant discloses a disability in their written candidature, they must be invited to an interview as long as the job is advertised. The employer is also obliged to involve the disability officer. Furthermore, it is very difficult to reject a disabled candidate who is comparable to his or her competitors in terms of qualifications [3].

It has been observed that many employers and department chairs do not appreciate the extra effort and are happy to choose the future employee independently, without having to worry about interference from the legal department, for example. Given the likelihood that an individual's selection is motivated by factors such as personality and qualifications rather than disability, it may be prudent to refrain from mentioning your disability in a written application.

During the probationary period, the legal protection available to disabled individuals against dismissal is contingent upon their ability to substantiate that the termination of their employment was attributable to their disability. This is a challenging proposition to substantiate, and thus, it is not advisable to assume a role in which one is likely to be swiftly dismissed.

In instances where an invitation is extended for an in-person interview, it is recommended to arrange for a job shadowing period, should there be mutual interest. Such an arrangement facilitates the assessment of whether the existing structural conditions present significant challenges. At the conclusion of a promising application process, the impairment should be mentioned, along with any necessary support. In the unfortunate event of a subsequent conflict within the team, the superior cannot claim ignorance regarding the constraints. It is often beneficial to demonstrate an openness to facing challenges, including night shifts, with which one is not yet familiar, and to vocalize the willingness to embrace it. Individuals who have previously held fulfilling roles can request that their previous supervisors provide contact information for their future superiors, a gesture that might foster trust.

18.8 In the Context of Professional Interactions

In the case of visible disabilities, the use of self-deprecating humor can serve to break the ice, and the individual can signal their openness to questions. It is preferable to respond to even the most silly questions than to have people talk behind your back. It is important to note that individuals may encounter recurrent exposure to comparisons due to the possibility of acquaintances having access to individuals who are presumed to possess similar limitations. It is appropriate to point out that individuals are unique and that disabilities manifest differently in different people. After all influenza, for instance, can manifest in a variety of ways, from relatively mild symptoms to severe complications.

In instances of open or semi-open discrimination from superiors, colleagues from other departments, or referrers, individuals have reported positive experiences of briefly highlighting these issues in a humorous manner, and if deemed necessary, hinting the legal context, such as "You're on very thin ice." In the event of recurrence, a simple smile and a retort such as "Oh, something new?" may be sufficient to deflect the initial reaction. However, should the matter persist or escalate, it is advisable to discreetly making the matter known to a superior of the offending individual, to ensure that some, at best appropriate, action is taken and to mitigate further difficulties.

Should a mood develop in the department that diminishes one's competence or commitment, not due to individual animosities, but rather due to your disability for which the individual is not responsible, such as the inability to cover 24-hour shifts or to work independently in angiography, it is advisable to seek out allies. An open, initially casual one-to-one discussion is recommended for this purpose. People who have experienced discrimination for other reasons are most likely to be supportive. In instances where bullying or bossing escalates, it is essential to approach the head of department in an objective manner and ask for support. It is important to note that not all senior managers are capable of taking responsibility for preventing discrimination in their own department. In such instances, it may be advisable to consider having a difficult conversation in the presence of the disability officer, who can offer support in attempting to effect positive change, or even resigning.

In the medical field, it has been observed that a propensity to seek opportunities for career progression may be associated with a willingness to transition between roles. While it might appear to be cowardly to leave in a state of emotional distress, it should be recognized that exposure to a toxic environment will not yield professional or personal development.

18.9 How to Enable and Promote a Team of Differently Abled Individuals: A Management Perspective

Irrespective of the presence of individuals with physical disabilities within the team, or the proactive decision to recruit a disabled individual, a substantial degree of influence can be exerted on the prevailing circumstances and the magnitude of the disability, particularly within the context of the entity operated.

A proactive approach to disability, with a focus on providing support, can create an environment where individuals feel more comfortable disclosing their needs and exploring potential solutions. Individuals with disabilities have often been managing their limitations for an extended period; therefore, it is advisable to inquire about past strategies that have proven effective. Individuals motivated to perform well are often willing to attempt a variety of strategies with the aim of optimizing their functionality within the team setting. These efforts should be greeted with appreciation, and it is essential to recognize that not all attempts may be successful. It should be emphasized to the employee that their ability to contribute and their competence are more important than their disability, especially as the impact of disabilities on work performance is frequently overstated [26].

In certain cases, it may be advantageous to promote specialization in specific areas, as this can potentially engender autonomy for those affected and alleviate them from the constant competition associated with physical demands.

It is incumbent upon managers to take responsibility in front of the team. When considering the integration of individuals with support needs within a team environment, it remains essential to articulate this objective in a transparent manner. There is evidence that teams exhibiting a high degree of diversity tend to demonstrate higher levels of productivity, satisfaction, and creativity [27]. However, it should be communicated that many, and not only those living with disabilities, require adjustments to the conditions in order to meet their needs [26]. It is recommendable to emphasize the aspiration for greater diversity and to express acceptance of the additional effort required to achieve it.

The development of a mission statement in conjunction with employees can serve to reflect their values in the design of the department, thereby ensuring that diversity is not perceived as an imposition.

One needs to acknowledge that inclusive practices can present challenges for all stakeholders; therefore, it is essential to heed the concerns of those who perceive inclusivity as a burdensome obligation [28].

The utilization of team coaching with an external coach who is disability-sensitive can also be beneficial in situations where there is significant discord within the team. Initial advice on this matter can be obtained from national organizations for the disabled, such as "Aktion Mensch" in Germany.

It is encouraging to note that there are numerous external funding opportunities available, including those specifically designed for conversion measures, employment assistance, and wage subsidies. However, these schemes are subject to local conditions. But in most cases, a company's disability officer will be very well informed and willing to offer consultation.

While the initial investment of time and energy to establish inclusive work environments can be substantial, it is generally observed to decrease quickly and substantially once implemented [28].

The potential benefits of inclusive work practices are manifold, including the cultivation of long-term loyalty among employees, an enhancement of team spirit, and the facilitation of trust and productivity [29].

Disclaimer Although most types of impairment, whether physical or mental, do not preclude a person from working in healthcare, at least as long as they have passed medical school, this chapter will focus on people with physical impairments. It is hoped that greater acceptance of a more diverse and inclusive society at large will eventually translate into less stigma around mental health conditions in the healthcare industry, so that we can learn more about and from these colleagues and include them in future discussions.

Bibliography

1. Dusel J. Die UN-Behindertenrechtskonvention Übereinkommen Über Die Rechte von Menschen Mit Behinderungen. https://www.behindertenbeauftragter.de/DE/AS/rechtliches/un-brk/un-brk-node.html. Accessed 12th April 2025.
2. Jochmaring J, York J. Inclusion opportunities of work 4.0? Employment realities of people with disabilities in Germany. Scand J Disabil Res. 2023;25(1):29–44. https://doi.org/10.16993/sjdr.896.
3. AGG. https://www.gesetze-im-internet.de/agg/. Accessed 14th April 2025.
4. statista. https://www.statista.com/statistics/1409050/inclusion-people-disabilities-workforce-germany/.
5. Andreas H, Christiane G. Education systems and inequalities: international comparisons. Policy Press; 2016.
6. Gréaux M, Moro MF, Kamenov K, Russell AM, Barrett D, Cieza A. Health equity for persons with disabilities: a global scoping review on barriers and interventions in healthcare services. Int J Equity Health. 2023;22(1) https://doi.org/10.1186/s12939-023-02035-w.
7. Kuper H, Azizatunnisa' L, Gatta DR, et al. Building disability-inclusive health systems. Lancet Public Health. 2024;9(5):e316–25. https://doi.org/10.1016/S2468-2667(24)00042-2.
8. Harker L. Unlocking the benefits of an inclusive health workforce diversifying Georgia's health workforce could expand access, improve care; 2016. https://www.gbpi.org.
9. Khuntia J, Ning X, Cascio W, Stacey R. Valuing diversity and inclusion in health care to equip the workforce: survey study and pathway analysis. JMIR Form Res. 2022;6(5) https://doi.org/10.2196/34808.
10. Stanford FC. The importance of diversity and inclusion in the healthcare workforce. J Natl Med Assoc. 2020;112(3):247–9. https://doi.org/10.1016/j.jnma.2020.03.014.
11. Kiradoo, Giriraj, Diversity, Equity, and Inclusion in the Workplace: Strategies for Achieving and Sustaining a Diverse Workforce (December 20, 2022). Advance Research in Social Science and Management. 2022. Edition 01, pp. 139–151, https://ssrn.com/abstract=4392136.
12. Ferdman BM, Deane BR, editors. Diversity at work: the practice of inclusion. Wiley; 2013. https://doi.org/10.1002/9781118764282.
13. Swartz TH, Palermo AGS, Masur SK, Aberg JA. The science and value of diversity: closing the gaps in our understanding of inclusion and diversity. J Infect Dis. 2019;220:S33–41. https://doi.org/10.1093/infdis/jiz174.
14. Lightfoote JB, Fielding JR, Deville C, et al. Improving diversity, inclusion, and representation in radiology and radiation oncology part 1: why these matter. J Am Coll Radiol. 2014;11(7):673–80. https://doi.org/10.1016/j.jacr.2014.03.007.
15. Habib H, Keller EJ. Disability in interventional radiology. Semin Intervent Radiol. 2021;38(4):500–3. https://doi.org/10.1055/s-0041-1735604.
16. Carr D, Namkung EH. Physical disability at work: how functional limitation affects perceived discrimination and interpersonal relationships in the workplace. J Health Soc Behav. 2021;62(4):545–61. https://doi.org/10.1177/00221465211023424.
17. van Beukering IE, Smits SJC, Janssens KME, et al. In what ways does health related stigma affect sustainable employment and Well-being at work? A systematic review. J Occup Rehabil. 2022;32(3):365–79. https://doi.org/10.1007/s10926-021-09998-z.
18. https://hbr.org/2024/11/research-the-stigma-disabled-people-face-during-negotiations. Accessed 12th April 2025.
19. Prizeman K, Weinstein N, McCabe C. Effects of mental health stigma on loneliness, social isolation, and relationships in young people with depression symptoms. BMC Psychiatry. 2023;23(1):527. https://doi.org/10.1186/s12888-023-04991-7.
20. Disabled People's Association & Institute of Policy Studies. Discrimination faced by people with disabilities at the workplace: A qualitative study. 2016. https://www.dpa.org.sg/wp-content/uploads/2018/07/Discrimination-Faced-by-People-with-Disabilities-at-the-Workplace-Study-1.pdf.

21. Shaw J, Wickenden M, Thompson S, Mader P. Achieving disability inclusive employment—are the current approaches deep enough? J Int Dev. 2022;34(5):942–63. https://doi.org/10.1002/jid.3692.
22. Brigham CR. AMA guides-sixth edition: evolving concepts, challenges and opportunities; 2011. https://www.impairment.com.
23. Taiwo OA, Cantley L. Impairment and disability evaluation: the role of the family physician. Am Fam Physician. 2008;77(12):1689–94. http://ecfr.gpoaccess.gov/cgi/t/text/text-idx?c=ecfr&sid=ace14df6f.
24. Perchik JD, Iheke JC, West JT, et al. Disruptive behavior: impact on diversity, equity, and inclusion (DEI) in radiology, from the AJR special series on DEI. Am J Roentgenol. 2023;221(2):163–70. https://doi.org/10.2214/AJR.22.28962.
25. https://ogletree.de/blog-posts/new-german-law-aims-to-promote-a-more-inclusive-labor-market/?lang=en. Accessed 13th April 2025.
26. Chumo I, Kabaria C, Mberu B. Social inclusion of persons with disability in employment: what would it take to socially support employed persons with disability in the labor market? Front Rehabil Sci. 2023:4. https://doi.org/10.3389/fresc.2023.1125129.
27. Turi JA, Khastoori S, Sorooshian S, Campbell N. Diversity impact on organizational performance: moderating and mediating role of diversity beliefs and leadership expertise. PLoS One. 2022;17(7 July) https://doi.org/10.1371/journal.pone.0270813.
28. Eshete SK, Birbirssa ZA. Strategic Human Resource Management (SHRM) in creating inclusive workplace: systematic review. SAGE Open. 2024;14(4):21582440241287668. https://doi.org/10.1177/21582440241287667.
29. Saxena A. Workforce diversity: a key to improve productivity. Procedia Econ Financ. 2014;11:76–85. https://doi.org/10.1016/s2212-5671(14)00178-6.

Addressing the Shortage of Specialists in Clinical Medicine and Radiology Through Healthcare Migration

19

Elif Can

19.1 Introduction

The global shortage of specialists in clinical medicine and radiology has reached a critical juncture, driven by factors such as aging populations, technological advancements, and the rising prevalence of complex medical conditions. Instrumental rationality reduces complex human identities to quantifiable outputs, obscuring the lived realities of marginalized groups [1]. This lens is particularly relevant in healthcare migration, where policies often fail to account for the intersectional challenges faced by professionals who navigate multiple axes of discrimination. By focusing solely on workforce numbers, systems risk perpetuating inequalities rather than addressing their root causes. This chapter explores healthcare migration as a potential solution to this shortage, analyzing the challenges and opportunities associated with integrating foreign-trained specialists into healthcare systems worldwide. WHO's Global Code of Practice on the International Recruitment of Health Personnel underscores the ethical dilemma of healthcare migration, emphasizing the need for fair recruitment practices that do not disproportionately drain resources from low- and middle-income countries [2].

It also highlights the role of radiology, particularly interventional radiology (IR), in addressing these shortages while discussing barriers, curriculum standardization, and the use of new Technologies to support integration efforts.

E. Can (✉)
Department of Diagnostic and Interventional Radiology, Medical Center University of Freiburg, Faculty of Medicine, University of Freiburg, Freiburg, Germany
e-mail: elif.can@uniklinik-freiburg.de

S. Keller-Yamamura, J. Yamamura (eds.), *Inclusive Radiology: Fostering Diversity and Equity in Academic and non-Academic Settings*,
https://doi.org/10.1007/978-3-032-05705-1_19

19.2 The Scope of the Problem

19.2.1 Global Demand for Specialists

The demand for specialized healthcare professionals continues to grow globally. According to the World Health Organization (WHO), there is an estimated shortfall of 18 million healthcare workers by 2030, primarily in low- and middle-income countries [2]. The Association of American Medical Colleges (AAMC) projects a shortage of 37,800–124,000 physicians by 2034, with up to 19,500 of these in medical specialties such as radiology [3]. Interventional radiology (IR) has evolved into an indispensable part of modern medicine, addressing conditions such as cancer, vascular diseases, and hepatobiliary conditions. These advancements require highly skilled professionals capable of utilizing state-of-the-art imaging technologies and delivering minimally invasive therapies [4]. However, training and recruiting sufficient specialists in IR has not kept pace with its rapid expansion, creating a gap that exacerbates healthcare inequalities.

In high-income countries such as the United States, Germany, and Japan, the demand for radiologists is expected to surpass supply in the coming years. Europe averages 13 radiologists per 100,000 population, while the United Kingdom has only 8.5 per 100,000, highlighting disparities that extend across the continent [3, 5–8].

The challenges extend beyond absolute numbers to include geographic distribution. Urban centers are often well-served, while rural areas face severe shortages of specialists. This imbalance disproportionately affects vulnerable populations who rely on public healthcare systems, particularly in remote regions where access to diagnostic imaging and interventional procedures is already limited [9].

19.2.2 Curriculum Variability and Credentialing Challenges

One critical issue in radiology is the inconsistency in training curricula across countries. While some regions emphasize a unified approach to diagnostics and interventions, others have fragmented systems that make it challenging for foreign-trained specialists to adapt. For example, European countries such as the United Kingdom have established comprehensive frameworks for IR training, but these standards often differ significantly from those in the United States, Latin America, or Asia, creating barriers for international professionals seeking recognition of their qualifications [4, 10, 11].

Discrepancies in imaging techniques, procedural protocols, and evaluation methods lead to inefficiencies and prolonged integration times for migrant specialists. Collaborative initiatives, such as the European Board of Radiology's efforts to harmonize training standards, offer promising pathways for addressing these challenges [12]. Standardizing diagnostic and interventional radiology curricula globally could facilitate credential recognition and reduce barriers for professionals wishing to work abroad [4, 13].

19.3 Migration Trends and Ethical Dilemmas

19.3.1 North–South Disparities

Migration trends often reflect inequities between the Global North and South. Countries in the Global North attract healthcare workers from the Global South due to better salaries, working conditions, and career advancement opportunities. Over one million people sought refuge in the EU in 2015, a fivefold increase from the year before... Many Member States are not implementing long-term plans or integration strategies, ensuring that they remain transit countries only [14]. For instance, approximately 25–32% of doctors in Australia, Canada, the United Kingdom, and the United States are international medical graduates (IMGs) who have trained in countries such as India, Pakistan, and sub-Saharan Africa. While this migration alleviates shortages in high-income countries, it exacerbates workforce deficits in resource-constrained regions [3, 6]. The EU's securitization policies in migration management have disproportionately impacted migrants from the Middle East, Africa, and Asia, reinforcing racial hierarchies of dominance and exploitation [14]. The ENAR Shadow Report (2015–2016) highlights that healthcare migration often exacerbates systemic inequalities, with high-income countries disproportionately benefiting from skilled professionals trained in low-resource settings. For example, approximately 25% of doctors in the United Kingdom were trained abroad, with significant contributions from South Asia and sub-Saharan Africa [14]. However, these migrations leave source countries with severe workforce deficits, creating ethical concerns about equitable healthcare access globally. The report underscores the importance of adhering to the WHO's Global Code of Practice on the International Recruitment of Health Personnel.

High-income countries often rely on healthcare workers from low-income regions, leading to inequities. For instance, 25–32% of doctors in countries like the United States and the United Kingdom are international medical graduates, exacerbating shortages in the Global South. Ethical recruitment policies, such as those outlined by the WHO, are necessary to address this imbalance [14]. Concerns arise when high-income countries actively recruit specialists from countries with critical workforce shortages. Addressing these disparities requires international collaboration to ensure equitable recruitment practices and support for healthcare development in source countries. Programs such as the WHO's Global Code of Practice on the International Recruitment of Health Personnel offer frameworks to mitigate these challenges, but enforcement and adherence remain inconsistent [2].

19.4 Structural Barriers and Discrimination

Migrant healthcare professionals frequently encounter structural discrimination in their host countries [14–20]. Structural violence, characterized by systemic inequalities embedded in institutional frameworks, perpetuates disparities and affects both professional integration and personal well-being [17, 21–23]. Discriminatory practices often manifest in unequal access to career advancement, resource allocation, and fair workloads [20, 24]. Can et al. (2022) conducted a survey of migrant healthcare professionals in Germany, finding that 58% reported experiencing discrimination in their work environments. Structural barriers, such as language difficulties and lack of mentorship, were cited as significant challenges to integration. Additionally, these professionals faced inequities in career progression, with only 20% feeling they had equal opportunities compared to their local counterparts. The study emphasizes the need for tailored onboarding programs and policy interventions to improve retention and job satisfaction [18].

Hattery et al. (2022) describe how intersectionality complicates the experiences of migrant healthcare professionals, particularly women of color. Black female doctors frequently encounter compounded discrimination based on both gender and race, impacting their access to leadership roles and career advancement opportunities. For instance, only 5% of surveyed minority women in leadership positions reported feeling adequately supported by their institutions. The study calls for organizational reforms, such as mentorship programs and intersectional diversity training, to address these disparities effectively [20].

Halley et al. (2018) revealed that physician mothers frequently face discrimination related to maternity leave, with 70% experiencing gender bias and 30% reporting harassment. These systemic barriers disproportionately affect migrant women physicians, who often lack access to support networks in their host countries. Addressing such disparities requires institutional policies that ensure equitable treatment and career progression opportunities for women balancing professional and caregiving responsibilities. Physician mothers revealed persistent gender discrimination, particularly around maternity leave policies and work–life balance. One respondent shared that “all part-time positions were held by women, yet a male physician in the same role earned 150% more.” Structural changes are needed to address these disparities [17].

Intersectionality adds another layer of complexity. Overlapping identities such as race, gender, and migration status can compound disadvantages [25]. Intersectional discrimination is prevalent globally, and addressing these nuanced challenges requires targeted policies that consider the interconnected nature of these identities [26]. In radiology, where leadership roles are predominantly held by men, women—especially those from minority backgrounds—face additional hurdles in advancing their career [26–29].

19.5 Leveraging Technology for Integration

19.5.1 Role of Large Language Models (LLMs)

Large language models (LLMs) have the potential to streamline the integration of migrant healthcare workers by providing real-time translations, localized medical guidelines, and reducing administrative burdens. LLMs like GPT-4 can play a pivotal role in overcoming language barriers, assisting with the translation of medical documentation, and offering real-time interpretation during clinical interactions [30–32]. These tools can significantly enhance communication between healthcare teams and migrant professionals, facilitating smoother integration into multidisciplinary environments [33]. Additionally, LLMs can be customized to provide localized medical guidelines and procedural norms, addressing regional differences in practice [34–36].

Integrating LLMs into radiology workflows could enable migrant specialists to rapidly adapt to new reporting standards, ensuring consistency in diagnostic accuracy. Such technologies also hold potential for reducing administrative burdens, allowing professionals to focus on patient care [37, 38]. Future advancements in AI could further refine these capabilities, providing tailored support for specific tasks, such as image analysis and procedural planning [39].

19.5.2 Telemedicine and Collaborative Platforms

Telemedicine and digital platforms can bridge gaps in training and professional development, enabling specialists from low-resource settings to gain exposure to advanced techniques and technologies. Virtual training programs and online knowledge-sharing networks can foster international collaboration, reducing barriers to skill acquisition [7, 9, 40]. For example, radiology departments in high-income countries could establish virtual mentorship programs to support migrant professionals and facilitate their integration into local healthcare systems. Telemedicine platforms and virtual mentorship programs have proven effective in bridging training gaps, particularly in resource-constrained settings. These tools enable migrant specialists to gain exposure to advanced techniques without the need for physical relocation.

19.6 Strategies for Integration and Equity

19.6.1 Institutional Support

Hospitals and healthcare systems must implement robust onboarding programs that include language training, cultural competency workshops, and mentor- and sponsorship [41, 42]. These initiatives can help migrant specialists navigate systemic challenges and integrate effectively into multidisciplinary teams. Racial discrimination in the labor market and housing sector continues to hinder integration efforts, as language proficiency is often used as a pretext for exclusion [14]. Mentorship programs tailored to women and minority healthcare professionals have been shown to improve retention rates by 30%, emphasizing the importance of targeted interventions in fostering an inclusive workplace [20]. Healthcare organizations should incorporate intersectionality into diversity training programs [43–45]. Intersectionality highlights how overlapping identities such as race, gender, and migration status exacerbate discrimination, requiring a nuanced approach to addressing these inequities [24]. Crenshaw (1989) argues that addressing the intersection of race and gender is crucial to understanding structural inequality, particularly in systems like healthcare that are fraught with implicit biases and systemic barriers [25]. Recognizing the unique challenges faced by professionals at the intersection of multiple identities can lead to more effective and inclusive workplace policies [5, 18, 19, 25, 46]. As Stuart Hall (2002) reminds us, racism is not a static construct but a dynamic, "floating signifier," capable of evolving in response to shifting societal structures. Addressing healthcare migration's challenges requires a similarly dynamic approach, one that actively dismantles these evolving biases through sustained institutional reforms, inclusive policies, and a commitment to equity at all levels [23]. Additionally, mentorship programs that connect migrant specialists with established professionals can help bridge gaps in understanding and foster a supportive environment. Implementing global initiatives, such as the International Network for Equity in Healthcare (INEH), can further promote equitable practices and foster a diverse healthcare workforce. Diverse research teams create unique opportunities for innovation but require intentional equity and inclusion efforts. Without this, diversity becomes a superficial checkbox rather than a meaningful change [20]. Hattery and colleagues quote, research shows that diverse teams are more creative but also experience higher levels of conflict. High-performing teams demonstrate better communication and greater satisfaction, even when working on complex tasks. These findings underscore the importance of actively supporting equity and inclusion within diverse teams to harness their full potential [20]. International recruitment practices must balance workforce needs with equitable support for healthcare development in source countries [2, 16, 47]. Strengthening ethical recruitment frameworks and investing in education and infrastructure in low-resource regions can create a more balanced global healthcare landscape. Bilateral agreements for workforce exchange and collaborative training programs can enhance mobility while ensuring sustainability. Efforts to standardize diagnostic and interventional radiology training programs could address inconsistencies and facilitate the global mobility of specialists [48]. Unified curricula would ensure that professionals meet consistent standards of practice, regardless of their country of origin [4, 12, 13, 49]. Such measures would also reduce the time required for credential recognition and improve workforce planning across borders. The European Training Curriculum for Radiology aims to harmonize training standards across member states, but significant variability remains, particularly in the integration of interventional radiology (IR) skills [12]. The Cardiovascular and Interventional Radiological Society of Europe (CIRSE) emphasizes the need for a unified syllabus for interventional radiology, arguing that standardized training can reduce the adaptation period for migrant specialists and ensure consistent patient care [4, 13]. A unified training curriculum for interventional radiology would not only facilitate global mobility for specialists but also ensure consistent standards of care, irrespective of geographic location.

19.7 Conclusion

Future efforts to address the global shortage of healthcare specialists must move beyond quantifiable metrics and embrace a holistic understanding of systemic inequities. Policies grounded in ethical recruitment, interdisciplinary innovation, and sustained global collaboration offer the potential to transform healthcare migration into a model of equity and resilience. Biases evolve with societal structures, necessitating a dynamic, adaptive approach to dismantling them. By centering the voices and experiences of historically marginalized groups, we can ensure that healthcare migration is not only a solution to workforce gaps but also a pathway toward a more inclusive and equitable global healthcare system. Inclusion exists only when historically excluded voices are centered, requiring researchers to engage in their own re-education about privilege and social inequities [20]. Healthcare migration is a viable solution to the global shortage of specialists in clinical medicine and radiology, but its success hinges on addressing structural and intersectional barriers. Labor market integration appears promising but often places undue responsibility on migrants, failing to address structural barriers such as racial discrimination, which significantly impacts employment opportunities for racialized individuals (ENAR Shadow Report, 2015–2016) [14]. By fostering inclusive and equitable workplaces, standardizing curricula, and leveraging technological advancements like LLMs, healthcare systems can attract and retain migrant professionals, ensuring sustainable growth in specialist care. Future research should explore the experiences of migrant specialists to inform targeted interventions and policy reforms. Expanding global collaboration on training and credentialing processes, while addressing ethical concerns and leveraging technology, could further enhance the efficiency and equity of healthcare migration. A truly international approach to healthcare migration can transform global healthcare delivery, ensuring that all regions have access to high-quality, specialized care.

References

1. Adorno TW, Horkheimer M. Dialectic of enlightenment. New York: Herder and Herder; 1972(1944).
2. Organization WH. WHO health workforce support and safeguards list 2023. Geneva: World Health Organization; 2023.

3. Dall TRR, Chakrabarti R, Ruttinger C, Zarek P, Parker O. The complexities of physician supply and demand: projections from 2021 to 2036. Washington, DC: AAMC by GlobalData Plc; 2024.
4. Morgan RA, Patel PJ, Binkert C, Tam A, (SIR) CaIRSoECatSoIR. Global statement defining interventional radiology-have we reached the tipping point? J Vasc Interv Radiol. 2024;47:1433.
5. Rhead RD, Chui Z, Bakolis I, Gazard B, Harwood H, MacCrimmon S, et al. Impact of workplace discrimination and harassment among National Health Service staff working in London trusts: results from the TIDES study. BJPsych Open. 2020;7(1):e10.
6. Observatory NRaH. Ethnic inequalities in healthcare: a rapid evidence review. February 2022.
7. Radiology ESo. Teleradiology in the European Union. Vienna: European Society of Radiology.
8. Pinto dos Santos D, Hempel JM, Kloeckner R, Düber C, Mildenberger P. Teleradiology - update 2014. Radiologe. 2014;54(5):487–90.
9. Hanna TN, Steenburg SD, Rosenkrantz AB, Pyatt RS, Duszak R, Friedberg EB. Emerging challenges and opportunities in the evolution of teleradiology. AJR Am J Roentgenol. 2020;215(6):1411–6.
10. Li S, Sun VH, Galla N, Salazar G, Lewis T, Ahmed M, et al. Gender-based survey analysis of research and mentoring in interventional radiology. J Vasc Interv Radiol. 2022;33(5):578–85.e3.
11. Grimm LJ, Lowell DA, Cater SW, Yoon SC. Differential motivations for pursuing diagnostic radiology by gender: implications for residency recruitment. Acad Radiol. 2017;24(10):1312–7.
12. (ESR) ESoR. European training curriculum for Subspecialisation in radiology: curriculum for the level III training programme (Subspecialisation beyond year 5). Vienna: European Society of Radiology (ESR); 2020.
13. Uberoi R, et al. European curriculum and syllabus for interventional radiology. 3rd ed. Vienna: Cardiovascular and Interventional Radiological Society of Europe (CIRSE); 2020.
14. Nwabuzo OaS, L. Racism and discrimination in the context of migration to Europe. European Network Against Racism Shadow Report 2015–2016. OECD; 2018. International migration outlook 2018. Technical report, OECD Publishing, Paris 2017.
15. Woodhams C, Williams M, Dacre J, Parnerkar I, Sharma M. Retrospective observational study of ethnicity-gender pay gaps among hospital and community health service doctors in England. BMJ Open. 2021;11(12):e051043.
16. Solomos J, Back L, British Sociological A. Racism and society. Basingstoke: Palgrave Macmillan; 1996.
17. Halley MC, Rustagi AS, Torres JS, Linos E, Plaut V, Mangurian C, et al. Physician mothers' experience of workplace discrimination: a qualitative analysis. BMJ. 2018;363:k4926.
18. Can E, Konrad CM, Khan-Gökkaya S, Molwitz I, Nawabi J, Yamamura J, et al. Foreign healthcare professionals in Germany: a questionnaire survey evaluating discrimination experiences and equal treatment at two large university hospitals. Healthcare (Basel). 2022;10(12)
19. Carr PL, Ash AS, Friedman RH, Szalacha L, Barnett RC, Palepu A, et al. Faculty perceptions of gender discrimination and sexual harassment in academic medicine. Ann Intern Med. 2000;132(11):889–96.
20. Hattery AJ, Smith E, Magnuson S, Monterrosa A, Kafonek K, Shaw C, Mhonde RD, Kanewske LC. Diversity, equity, and inclusion in research teams: the good, the bad, and the ugly. In: Race and Justice, vol. 12. SAGE Publications; 2022. p. 505–30.
21. Hamed S, Thapar-Björkert S, Bradby H, Ahlberg BM. Racism in European health care: structural violence and beyond. Qual Health Res. 2020;30(11):1662–73.
22. Gopal DP, Rao M. Playing hide and seek with structural racism. BMJ. 2021;373:n988.
23. Hall S. Stuart Hall: race, the floating signifier. Northampton: Media Education Foundation; 2002.
24. Likupe G. Experiences of African nurses and the perception of their managers in the NHS. J Nurs Manag. 2015;23(2):231–41.
25. Crenshaw K, Fletcher R. Demarginalizing the intersection of race and sex: a black feminist critique of antidiscrimination doctrine, feminist theory and anti-racist politics. In: Feminist legal theories. Routledge.

26. Martinez NE. Women in radiation: a brief discussion of the intersectionality of race and gender. J Radiol Prot. 2021;41(3):590.
27. Kubik-Huch RA, Vilgrain V, Krestin GP, Reiser MF, Attenberger UI, Muellner AU, et al. Women in radiology: gender diversity is not a metric-it is a tool for excellence. Eur Radiol. 2020;30(3):1644–52.
28. Schueller-Weidekamm C, Kautzky-Willer A. Challenges of work-life balance for women physicians/mothers working in leadership positions. Gend Med. 2012;9(4):244–50.
29. Baker SR, Barry M, Chaudhry H, Hubbi B. Women as radiologists: are there barriers to entry and advancement? J Am Coll Radiol. 2006;3(2):131–4.
30. Aerts A, Bogdan-Martin D. Leveraging data and AI to deliver on the promise of digital health. Int J Med Inform. 2021;150:104456.
31. Hazarika I. Artificial intelligence: opportunities and implications for the health workforce. Int Health. 2020;12(4):241–5.
32. Katal S, York B, Gholamrezanezhad A. AI in radiology: from promise to practice - a guide to effective integration. Eur J Radiol. 2024;181:111798.
33. de Margerie-Mellon C. Leveraging artificial intelligence in radiology education: challenges and opportunities. Eur Radiol. 2023;33(11):8239–40.
34. Gomez-Cabello CA, Borna S, Pressman S, Haider SA, Haider CR, Forte AJ. Artificial-intelligence-based clinical decision support systems in primary care: a scoping review of current clinical implementations. Eur J Investig Health Psychol Educ. 2024;14(3):685–98.
35. Mohsen F, Ali H, El Hajj N, Shah Z. Artificial intelligence-based methods for fusion of electronic health records and imaging data. Sci Rep. 2022;12(1):17981.
36. Can E, Uller W, Vogt K, Doppler MC, Busch F, Bayerl N, et al. Large language models for simplified interventional radiology reports: a comparative analysis. Acad Radiol. 2024;32:888.
37. Fawzy NA, Tahir MJ, Saeed A, Ghosheh MJ, Alsheikh T, Ahmed A, et al. Incidence and factors associated with burnout in radiologists: a systematic review. Eur J Radiol Open. 2023;11:100530.
38. Molwitz I. Joy at work: how to build a happy and resilient next generation of radiologists. Eur Radiol. 2024;34(1):692–4.
39. Pinto Dos Santos D, Baeßler B. Big data, artificial intelligence, and structured reporting. Eur Radiol Exp. 2018;2(1):42.
40. Özmen MN, Dicle O, Şenol U, Aydıngöz Ü. TSR guidelines for the practice of teleradiology: 2021 update. Diagn Interv Radiol. 2021;27(4):504–10.
41. Deitte LA, McGinty GB, Canon CL, Omary RA, Johnson PT, Slanetz PJ. Shifting from mentorship to sponsorship-a game changer! J Am Coll Radiol. 2019;16(4 Pt A):498–500.
42. Martinez S, Araj J, Reid S, Rodriguez J, Nguyen M, Pinto DB, et al. Allyship in residency: an introductory module on medical Allyship for graduate medical trainees. MedEdPORTAL. 2021;17:11200.
43. Johnson J, Cameron L, Mitchinson L, Parmar M, Opio-Te G, Louch G, et al. An investigation into the relationships between bullying, discrimination, burnout and patient safety in nurses and midwives: is burnout a mediator? J Res Nurs. 2019;24(8):604–19.
44. Shore LM, Chung BG. Inclusion as a multi-level concept. Curr Opin Psychol. 2024;60:101910.
45. Lightfoote JB, Fielding JR, Deville C, Gunderman RB, Morgan GN, Pandharipande PV, et al. Improving diversity, inclusion, and representation in radiology and radiation oncology part 1: why these matter. J Am Coll Radiol. 2014;11(7):673–80.
46. Sellers RM, Shelton JN. The role of racial identity in perceived racial discrimination. J Pers Soc Psychol. 2003;84(5):1079–92.
47. Hall S. Cultural identity and diaspora; 2005.
48. Kelly AM, Mullan PB. Designing a curriculum for professionalism and ethics within radiology: identifying challenges and expectations. Acad Radiol. 2018;25(5):610–8.
49. Ullrich L, Uller W, Frisch A. Interventional radiology - training and career opportunities. Radiologie (Heidelb). 2024;65(1):47–51.

MIX
Papier aus verantwortungsvollen Quellen
Paper from responsible sources
FSC® C105338

If you have any concerns about our products,
you can contact us on
ProductSafety@springernature.com

In case Publisher is established outside the EU,
the EU authorized representative is:
Springer Nature Customer Service Center GmbH
Europaplatz 3, 69115 Heidelberg, Germany

Printed by Libri Plureos GmbH
in Hamburg, Germany